Meditation for immortality of the soul

Dedication

This book, "Meditation for Immortality of the Soul," is dedicated to the countless seekers who have embarked on their own spiritual journeys, bravely facing life's challenges with courage and unwavering faith. It is dedicated to those who have found solace and strength in the practice of meditation, transforming their lives and inspiring others to follow their path. This work is a testament to the resilience of the human spirit, the unwavering pursuit of self-discovery, and the enduring belief in the potential for inner peace and spiritual liberation. It is dedicated to those who dare to dream beyond the confines of the physical world, seeking a deeper understanding of their true selves and the boundless possibilities that lie beyond. This dedication extends to those who have shown kindness, compassion, and unwavering support on the path towards enlightenment, serving as guiding lights on the journey. It is with deep gratitude and heartfelt appreciation that I dedicate this book to every soul who yearns for a deeper connection to their essence, a life overflowing with purpose and meaning, a journey beyond the physical realm towards the immortality of the soul. May this book serve as a beacon, guiding you towards your own unique path of spiritual awakening and the realization of your boundless potential, a pathway towards inner peace and the eternal spirit within. This is a dedication to the relentless pursuit of truth, the unshakeable belief in the power of the human spirit, and the transformative potential of the human heart. To all who seek truth, wisdom, and lasting peace, this book is for you.

Preface

The journey to spiritual enlightenment is a deeply personal one, a path unique to each individual soul. Yet, within the vast tapestry of human experience, we discover common threads, shared experiences, and universal truths that connect us all. This book, "Meditation for Immortality of the Soul," emerges from a profound appreciation for this universal human yearning—the desire for deeper meaning, inner peace, and a connection to something greater than ourselves. It's a testament to the power of meditation as a transformative tool, not merely a relaxation technique, but a pathway to unlock our full potential, to navigate life's challenges with grace, and to cultivate a life of profound purpose and lasting fulfillment. Through the pages that follow, you will discover practical techniques, insightful wisdom, and empowering practices designed to guide you on your own personal journey. This is not just a guide to meditation; it is a guide to understanding your innate connection to the universe, to unlocking the wisdom within, and to fostering a life that resonates with authenticity, joy, and boundless love. My intention is to offer a supportive and encouraging voice, a guide to help you navigate this transformative process. Remember that the journey is the destination. The process of self-discovery and growth is a continuous unfolding, a testament to the ever-evolving nature of the human spirit. Embrace each step, honor each experience, and allow yourself the time and space to cultivate a deep and meaningful relationship with your own inner being. With unwavering dedication, let us embark on this enriching and enlightening journey together. May this book illuminate your path and guide you towards the life you were meant to live – a life of purpose, meaning, and the boundless potential of the soul.

Introduction

For millennia, humanity has sought the secrets to longevity, both in the physical and spiritual realms. While scientific advancements continue to extend our lifespans, a deeper yearning persists—a desire to transcend the limitations of the physical body and experience a form of immortality. This book, "Meditation for Immortality of the Soul," explores the powerful connection between meditation, spiritual growth, and the profound experience of lasting fulfillment. It proposes that true longevity extends far beyond the physical; it is a journey of self-discovery, a deepening of our connection to our inner selves, and an expansion of our consciousness beyond the confines of our physical existence. Through the practice of meditation, we can cultivate inner peace, enhance our vitality, and strengthen our connection to a higher power. The techniques outlined within these pages are not merely exercises for relaxation; they are tools for transformation, enabling us to navigate life's challenges with greater grace and resilience, to foster healthier relationships, and to cultivate a profound sense of purpose. This book is not about escaping life; it is about embracing it more fully. It is about discovering the boundless potential within each of us to live a life of profound meaning, joy, and connection—a life that transcends the boundaries of the physical and extends into the realm of the eternal. It is a journey of self-discovery, a journey of self-mastery, and a journey towards a state of being that embraces the fullness of life, both physical and spiritual, ultimately leading towards a profound understanding of what it truly means to be alive, fully and vibrantly, extending into the boundless realm of the spirit. This is an invitation to embark on a transformative journey – a journey towards the immortality of the soul.

Understanding the Interconnectedness of Mind Body and Spirit

The journey to spiritual enlightenment is not a linear path, but a holistic exploration of self. It's a profound understanding that our mind, body, and spirit are inextricably interwoven, a vibrant tapestry where each thread influences the others. Ignoring this fundamental interconnectedness is akin to attempting to mend a torn tapestry by focusing only on one thread—the result is inevitably incomplete and fragile. This chapter lays the groundwork for understanding this intricate relationship, preparing you for the transformative power of meditation.

Our modern world often compartmentalizes our well-being, separating the physical from the mental and the spiritual. We visit doctors for physical ailments, therapists for emotional distress, and perhaps a religious leader for spiritual guidance. While these approaches can be helpful, they often fail to address the root cause of imbalance, the underlying disharmony within the interconnected whole. True well-being, however, arises from a harmonious interplay of mind, body, and spirit. When one area suffers, the others inevitably follow suit. Chronic stress, for example, not only impacts our mental state, leading to anxiety and depression, but also manifests physically through headaches, digestive issues, and a weakened immune system. Similarly, neglecting our spiritual needs – our connection to something larger than ourselves – can leave us feeling empty and unfulfilled, regardless of our physical and mental health.

The concept of "prana," or life force, is central to understanding this interconnectedness. Prana is the vital energy that animates all living beings. In Ayurvedic tradition, prana is considered the life-giving breath, the essence that flows through our bodies, fueling our physical functions, emotions, and thoughts. When prana flows freely and unobstructed, we experience vitality, energy, and a sense of well-being. Conversely, blockages in the flow of prana can manifest as illness, fatigue, and emotional stagnation. Meditation, therefore, acts as a conduit, clearing blockages, harmonizing the flow of prana, and cultivating a state of vibrant health and longevity.

Think of your body as a complex machine, requiring energy to function optimally. This energy, in part, is derived from the food we eat and the oxygen we breathe. But the efficient utilization of this energy is also dependent on the mental and emotional landscape. Constant worry, stress, and negativity create internal chaos, disrupting the smooth flow of energy. This creates a vicious cycle: the disruption of energy flow results in fatigue, which further exacerbates negativity and worry. This is where meditation steps in, acting as a regulator, helping to restore a balanced flow of energy. Through focused practices, we learn to calm the mind's turbulence, allowing the body to utilize energy more efficiently, fostering a state of well-being and increasing vitality.

Consider the limitations of a purely physical approach to well-being. We might diligently exercise, consume a nutritious diet, and receive regular medical checkups. Yet, if our mental and spiritual well-being are neglected, we may still struggle with chronic stress, anxiety, or a lack of purpose. The body, without the support of a calm mind and a nourished spirit, will only achieve a limited level of health and vitality. A holistic perspective, on the other hand, acknowledges the intricate dance between mind, body, and spirit, recognizing that true well-being is a symphony of harmonious interplay, not a collection of individual parts. It is a journey of self-discovery, leading to a profound understanding of the interconnections between our internal world and external reality.

To illustrate this principle, let's consider the experience of grief. The death of a loved one can have a profound impact on all three aspects of our being. Physically, we may experience fatigue, loss of appetite, or even physical illness. Mentally, we might experience overwhelming sadness, anxiety, and difficulty concentrating. Spiritually, we might question our beliefs, our sense of purpose, and our connection to something larger than ourselves. Traditional Western medicine might address the physical symptoms, psychotherapy might offer support for mental anguish, but addressing the spiritual void requires a different approach—a shift in perspective, a reconnection with inner peace, and a recognition of the enduring nature of the spirit. Meditation provides the tools to navigate these multifaceted challenges. It helps us to process our emotions, find solace in the present moment, and rediscover our inner strength and resilience. By addressing the mind, body, and spirit simultaneously, we can find a pathway to healing and wholeness.

Another example is the impact of chronic stress. The relentless demands of modern life often leave us feeling overwhelmed and depleted. This stress takes a toll not only on our mental health, leading to anxiety and depression, but also on our physical health, increasing the risk of heart disease, weakened immunity, and various other ailments. Spiritual neglect, in the form of a lack of connection to a higher purpose or a sense of meaning, often exacerbates the situation. Through meditation, we can learn to manage stress effectively, cultivating inner peace and resilience. We learn to observe our thoughts and emotions without judgment, gently releasing tension and finding a sense of calm amidst the chaos. This, in turn, has a positive impact on both our physical and mental well-being. Meditation strengthens our capacity to handle stress, to find moments of tranquility even in the midst of life's storms.

Understanding this holistic approach is crucial for embarking on the journey to spiritual enlightenment. It is not merely a pursuit of intellectual knowledge, but a profound transformation of our being – a shift from fragmentation to integration, from imbalance to harmony. This fundamental shift in perspective is the foundation upon which we build a life of vitality, purpose, and lasting well-being, a life that transcends the limitations of the physical realm and touches upon the immortality of the soul. The following sections will guide you through practical techniques to cultivate this harmony, using meditation as the primary tool to unlock your inherent potential. We will explore the power of breathwork, mindfulness, visualization, and advanced meditation practices, all designed to strengthen the connection between mind, body, and spirit. This interconnectedness is not just a concept, it is the very essence of who you are, waiting to be discovered and nurtured. The journey begins with recognizing this profound truth.

Breathwork and Mindfulness

The path to spiritual enlightenment, as we've begun to explore, is a journey of integration—a harmonious blending of mind, body, and spirit. Meditation acts as the vehicle for this journey, a tool to cultivate this vital connection and unlock the inherent potential within. Before we delve into more advanced techniques, it's essential to establish a strong foundation, a solid base upon which to build our meditative practice. This foundation is built upon two pillars: breathwork and mindfulness. These seemingly simple practices are, in reality, powerful keys to unlocking inner peace and accessing deeper states of consciousness.

Breathwork, the conscious control of our respiration, is often overlooked in our daily lives. We breathe automatically, unconsciously, rarely paying attention to the rhythm and depth of our breath. Yet, our breath is the bridge connecting our physical and spiritual selves. It's the life force, the subtle energy that animates our bodies and fuels our consciousness. By learning to consciously control our breath, we gain a direct pathway to influencing our mental and emotional states.

One of the simplest yet most effective breathing techniques is the diaphragmatic, or belly, breath. This involves consciously expanding the abdomen as you inhale, feeling the breath fill your lower lungs. As you exhale, gently contract your abdomen, allowing the breath to release completely. This technique engages the diaphragm, the primary muscle of respiration, promoting deeper, more rhythmic breathing. Try this exercise now:

Find a comfortable position, either sitting or lying down. Close your eyes gently. Bring your attention to your breath. Notice the natural rhythm of your inhalations and exhalations. Don't try to change anything, simply observe. Now, place one hand on your chest and the other on your abdomen. Inhale slowly and deeply through your nose, feeling your abdomen rise as your lungs fill with air. Your chest should remain relatively still. Exhale slowly through your mouth, feeling your abdomen gently contract. Continue this practice for 5-10 minutes, focusing solely on the sensation of your breath. Notice how your mind begins to quiet, how tension melts away with each exhale.

Beyond the simple diaphragmatic breath, there are countless other breathwork techniques. Alternate nostril breathing (Nadi Shodhana), for example, involves alternately closing one nostril and breathing through the other, balancing the flow of energy within the body. Ujjayi breath, or "ocean breath," involves a gentle constriction in the throat, creating a soft, hissing sound as you breathe. Each of these techniques offers unique benefits, affecting different aspects of our energy system and mental state. Experiment with different techniques to discover what resonates most with you. The key is consistency and mindful attention.

Mindfulness, the second pillar of our foundation, is the practice of paying attention to the present moment without judgment. It's about cultivating a state of awareness where we are fully present in our experience, observing our thoughts, feelings, and sensations without getting carried away by them. This ability to observe without judgment is crucial for breaking free from the cycle of reactive thinking and emotional turmoil that often keeps us from accessing our inner peace.

Many find it challenging to maintain focus on the present. Our minds are naturally prone to wandering, jumping from thought to thought, often dwelling on past regrets or future anxieties. Mindfulness is the art of gently guiding our attention back to the present when our minds wander, without self-criticism. This gentle redirection is key. It's not about suppressing thoughts or emotions, but about observing them with a detached, compassionate awareness.

A simple mindfulness exercise involves focusing on a single sensory experience. This could be the feeling of your breath against your skin, the sounds around you, or the sensations in your body. Choose one sensory input and focus your attention on it for a few minutes. When your mind wanders (and it will!), simply acknowledge the wandering thought without judgment and gently redirect your attention back to your chosen sensory experience.

Consider the following example: you might focus on the taste of a piece of fruit. Really savor it. Pay attention to its texture, its sweetness, its subtle nuances. Notice how your body responds to the flavors. Every time your mind drifts, gently guide it back to the fruit, acknowledging the wandering thoughts without dwelling on them.

This seemingly simple exercise is a powerful way to cultivate present moment awareness. It trains your mind to focus, to resist the allure of distraction. This focused attention is a fundamental skill in meditation, allowing you to deepen your practice and access deeper states of consciousness.

The combination of breathwork and mindfulness forms the bedrock of our meditative practice. These two pillars support the deeper exploration of our inner landscape, providing a stable platform for accessing higher states of being.

Mastering these basic techniques will not only calm your mind and reduce stress, but also lay the foundation for a more profound and transformative meditative experience.

Consider the body scan meditation. This is a form of mindfulness meditation, building upon the foundations of breathwork. Find a comfortable position, lying down is usually ideal. Begin with your breath, the gentle rhythm of inhalations and exhalations, noticing the sensation of the breath in your nostrils, your chest, your abdomen. As you settle into the rhythm, begin to bring your awareness to your body, starting with your toes. Notice any sensations— tingling, warmth, pressure, coolness—without judgment. Simply observe. Slowly move your awareness up your body, paying attention to each part—your feet, ankles, calves, knees, thighs, hips, abdomen, back, chest, shoulders, arms, hands, fingers, neck, face, head. Allow yourself to fully feel each part of your body, releasing any tension or holding you might find. As you scan your body, your breath acts as an anchor, guiding you back to the present moment whenever your mind wanders.

The integration of breathwork and mindfulness is not a passive process; it requires consistent effort and dedicated practice. Begin with short sessions, perhaps just five to ten minutes daily. As your comfort level increases, gradually lengthen your practice. The key is to make it a consistent part of your daily routine, creating a sacred space for inner reflection and self-discovery. The journey to spiritual enlightenment is a marathon, not a sprint. Consistent practice, even in small increments, yields remarkable results.

It's also crucial to approach these practices with kindness and compassion. There will be moments of frustration, moments where your mind resists staying present. This is perfectly normal. Do not judge yourself harshly for these moments.

Acknowledge them with compassion, gently redirect your attention back to your breath and your body, and continue the practice. The goal is not perfection, but progress. Each session, no matter how short or seemingly imperfect, is a step forward on your journey.

Remember, the journey to spiritual enlightenment is not solely about achieving a particular state of being; it's about the ongoing process of self-discovery, self-acceptance, and self-transformation. Breathwork and mindfulness provide the tools for this transformative process, allowing you to cultivate inner peace, increase self-awareness, and connect more deeply with your true self—the essence of your being that transcends the limitations of the physical realm, reaching towards the immortality of your soul. The path unfolds gradually, with each breath, each mindful moment, bringing you closer to the profound understanding and liberation that awaits. Embrace the journey, trust the process, and allow yourself to be transformed.

Detoxifying the Mind and Body

The journey toward spiritual enlightenment is not merely a mental exercise; it's a holistic endeavor encompassing the entirety of our being. Just as a sculptor carefully chisels away at excess stone to reveal the masterpiece within, so too must we refine our minds and bodies, releasing the impurities that obscure our inner light. This process of purification, of cultivating inner purity, is a crucial step in our ascent towards a higher state of consciousness. It's about creating a sanctuary within, a space of clarity and calm where the divine can reside.

Our minds, like cluttered attics, often accumulate a vast array of negative emotions, limiting beliefs, and unhealthy patterns. These mental toxins, if left unchecked, can poison our spiritual growth, hindering our ability to connect with our true selves and the universal consciousness. To counteract this, we must engage in a conscious effort to detoxify our minds. This begins with mindful awareness – observing our thoughts without judgment. Notice the patterns that emerge, the recurring anxieties, the self-critical voices. By simply witnessing these patterns, we begin to detach from them, lessening their power over us.

One powerful technique is the practice of meditation itself. Through focused attention on the breath or a mantra, we can quiet the incessant chatter of the mind, creating a space of stillness where these negative thoughts lose their potency. Imagine the mind as a turbulent sea; meditation is the anchor, grounding us in the present moment, allowing the waves of negativity to subside. Regular meditation, even for short periods, can dramatically transform the mental landscape, fostering a sense of inner peace and clarity.

Beyond meditation, journaling can be a profound tool for mental detoxification. Writing down our thoughts and emotions allows us to externalize them, bringing them into the light of awareness. This act of self-expression can be incredibly cathartic, releasing pent-up negativity and creating space for positive growth. Don't worry about grammar or style; simply allow the words to flow freely, expressing whatever arises without judgment.

Furthermore, the practice of forgiveness plays a vital role in mental purification. Holding onto resentment and anger only serves to poison our own energy field. Forgiveness, however, isn't about condoning harmful actions; it's about releasing the negativity that binds us to the past, freeing ourselves from its grip. Forgiving others, and even more importantly, forgiving ourselves, allows us to move forward with lightness and grace. This process can be facilitated through meditation, visualization, or simply through quiet reflection.

The body, too, requires attention in our pursuit of inner purity. What we consume directly influences our energy levels, our mental clarity, and our overall well-being. Mindful eating, therefore, becomes a spiritual practice. Pay close attention to the food you consume, choosing whole, unprocessed foods that nourish your body and spirit. Appreciate the energy that is transferred from the earth to your body in the form of nutrients. Cultivating awareness of our choices and understanding their impact shifts the simple act of eating into something far deeper.

Avoid excessive consumption of processed foods, sugar, caffeine, and alcohol. These substances can disrupt the delicate balance of the body and mind, leading to energy imbalances and mental fogginess. Instead, focus on nourishing your body with fresh fruits, vegetables, whole grains, and lean protein. Listen to your body's signals, eating mindfully and with appreciation.

Physical exercise also plays a vital role in the process of physical and mental purification. Exercise is more than just physical conditioning; it's a pathway to releasing stagnant energy, both physical and emotional. Regular movement, whether through yoga, walking, running, or any other activity that you enjoy, helps to clear blockages, improving circulation and stimulating the flow of life force energy throughout the body. This increased energy flow contributes to a heightened sense of vitality and clarity.

Yoga, in particular, is a powerful tool for physical and spiritual purification. The postures, or asanas, help to strengthen and stretch the body, while the breathing techniques, or pranayama, cultivate a deeper connection with the breath and promote a sense of calm and inner peace. The meditative aspect of yoga further enhances its ability to purify the body and mind, creating a holistic practice that enhances both physical and spiritual well-being.

Beyond physical exercise and diet, consider incorporating practices for emotional cleansing. These can include spending time in nature, listening to soothing music, engaging in creative expression, or practicing forgiveness techniques already mentioned. Anything that promotes a sense of peace and tranquility can contribute to the process of emotional detoxification, allowing you to release pent-up emotions and create a more balanced emotional state. Engaging in activities that bring you joy and cultivate a sense of inner peace will greatly support your spiritual journey.

These practices—mindful eating, regular exercise, emotional cleansing, and meditation—are not isolated actions; they are interconnected aspects of a holistic approach to spiritual growth. They work synergistically, creating a powerful synergy that elevates the quality of your life and deepens your connection to your inner self. The refinement of body and mind creates a more receptive vessel for spiritual experiences, allowing you to enter deeper meditative states and experience a greater sense of clarity and connection.

Remember, this journey is not a race; it's a process of gradual refinement. Be patient with yourself, celebrate your progress, and don't be discouraged by setbacks. Each step you take, no matter how small, brings you closer to your ultimate goal: a state of inner purity, a connection with your higher self, and the realization of your spiritual potential. The purification process is ongoing, a lifelong commitment to nurturing your body, mind, and spirit. Embrace the journey, and the path to enlightenment will naturally unfold. The path to immortality of the soul begins with the conscious purification of the physical and mental vessels that house it.

As you progress on your journey, notice how the quality of your meditation deepens. As you cleanse the mental and physical clutter, your mind becomes clearer, more focused, and more receptive to the subtle energies of the spiritual realm. The stillness you achieve in meditation will be profound, allowing you to access deeper levels of consciousness and experience states of profound peace and joy. This heightened clarity and inner peace will extend beyond your meditation practice, impacting every aspect of your life – your relationships, your work, and your overall sense of well-being. You'll find that you navigate challenges with greater ease, responding to life's ups and downs with a sense of groundedness and resilience.

Cultivating inner purity is not merely a step towards spiritual enlightenment; it's an essential aspect of living a fulfilling and meaningful life. It's a commitment to self-care, self-respect, and self-discovery. It's a journey of continuous growth and refinement, a pathway to unlocking the boundless potential within. Embrace the process; it is a testament to your commitment to your own spiritual evolution and a vital step on the path to the immortality of your soul. Through diligent practice and unwavering commitment, you will discover a profound sense of inner peace, clarity, and connection to something far greater than yourself. The path towards spiritual enlightenment is a marathon, not a sprint. Be patient with yourself and enjoy the journey.

Harnessing the Power of Visualization and Intention Setting

Building upon the foundation of inner purity and mindful awareness established in the previous chapter, we now embark on a journey into the potent realms of visualization and intention setting. These are not mere fanciful exercises; they are powerful tools that, when integrated into your meditative practice, can accelerate your spiritual growth and manifest your deepest desires. Think of visualization as sculpting your reality, chiseling away at limiting beliefs and shaping a life aligned with your soul's purpose. Intention setting is the blueprint, the guiding principle that directs the energy of your visualization, ensuring your efforts are focused and effective.

The power of visualization lies in its ability to bypass the critical, analytical mind and directly access the subconscious. Your subconscious mind, a vast repository of untapped potential, readily accepts and acts upon the images and feelings you consistently feed it. When you vividly visualize a desired outcome – whether it's improved health, a fulfilling career, a loving relationship, or a deeper connection to the divine – you are, in essence, programming your subconscious to work towards that reality. This is not about wishful thinking; it's about harnessing the innate power of your mind to shape your experience.

Imagine, for instance, visualizing yourself radiating vibrant health. Don't just see a healthy body; feel the energy flowing through you, the lightness in your step, the vitality in your being. Engage all your senses: the feel of fresh air on your skin, the taste of nourishing food, the strength in your muscles. The more vivid and emotionally resonant your visualization, the more powerful its effect on your subconscious. This is not a passive activity; it requires active engagement, a conscious effort to create a realistic and compelling mental picture.

Similarly, visualize achieving a specific professional goal. See yourself confidently presenting a successful project, receiving accolades for your achievements, experiencing the satisfaction of a job well done. Feel the sense of accomplishment, the pride in your work, the financial security it brings. The key is to engage your emotions, to feel the joy and fulfillment associated with the achievement. This emotional resonance amplifies the power of your visualization, making it a more effective tool for manifestation.

The practice of intention setting complements visualization by providing a clear direction for your mental energy. Before you begin visualizing, clearly articulate your intention. What specific outcome are you aiming for? Be precise and unambiguous. Avoid vague statements like "I want to be happy." Instead, define happiness in concrete terms: "I intend to cultivate a deep sense of inner peace and contentment, radiating love and joy in all my interactions." The more specific and measurable your intention, the clearer the path for your subconscious to follow.

Align your intentions with a higher purpose. Consider how your desired outcome contributes to your spiritual growth and aligns with your values. For example, if your intention is to achieve financial success, ask yourself: how will this success enable me to serve others, contribute to the well-being of my community, or further my spiritual journey? By aligning your intentions with a higher purpose, you infuse them with a deeper meaning and increase the likelihood of their manifestation.

The process of visualization and intention setting is most effective when integrated into your meditative practice. Find a quiet space, close your eyes, and begin by focusing on your breath. Allow your body to relax, your mind to quieten. Once you've achieved a state of deep relaxation, begin visualizing your desired outcome with clarity and intensity. Simultaneously, hold your intention firmly in your mind, reinforcing its power with each breath.

Remember, manifestation is not a quick fix; it's a gradual process that requires consistent effort and unwavering faith. Just as a sculptor patiently chisels away at stone to reveal the masterpiece within, you must patiently nurture your visualization and intention setting practice, allowing it to gradually transform your thoughts, emotions, and ultimately, your reality. Do not be discouraged by setbacks. View them as opportunities for growth and refinement, chances to reassess your intentions and refine your approach.

Consider journaling as a complementary practice. Regularly write down your intentions, visualizing your desired outcomes and reflecting on your progress. This reinforces your commitment and provides a space for self-reflection and adjustment. Note any obstacles you encounter and strategize how to overcome them. Celebrate your successes, however small, and use them to fuel your motivation.

The integration of visualization and intention setting into a broader spiritual practice is crucial. It's not enough to simply visualize success; you must also cultivate the inner qualities necessary to achieve it – discipline, perseverance, compassion, and a commitment to personal growth. Your spiritual journey is a holistic endeavor, and the tools of visualization and intention setting are but two instruments in a larger orchestra.

Let's delve into specific examples. Imagine you're struggling with a chronic health condition. Instead of focusing on the limitations imposed by your illness, visualize yourself radiating vibrant health and vitality. See your body healing, feel your energy levels rising, experience the joy of physical well-being. Simultaneously, set the intention to actively participate in your healing process. This might involve making healthy lifestyle choices, seeking professional medical assistance, and cultivating a positive mental attitude. Remember, visualization and intention setting work best in conjunction with practical action.

Another example: you're striving for professional success. Visualize yourself confidently presenting your ideas, receiving positive feedback, and achieving your career goals. Feel the satisfaction of accomplishment, the financial security, and the recognition of your hard work. Set the intention to work diligently, to hone your skills, and to network with others in your field. Remember to focus not only on the external outcome but also on the internal growth and development necessary to achieve it.

Ultimately, the power of visualization and intention setting lies in their ability to connect you with your inner wisdom and guide you towards a life that is both meaningful and fulfilling. By aligning your desires with your higher purpose, you create a ripple effect that extends beyond your personal life, positively impacting the world around you. This is a journey of continuous self-discovery, a process of refining your intentions and refining your vision, constantly striving towards a greater alignment between your inner world and your outer reality. Remember, the immortality of the soul is not merely an abstract concept; it's the realization of your full potential, a life lived with purpose, passion, and

unwavering faith in the power of your own mind and spirit.
The journey continues. Embrace the power within you.

Advanced Meditation Techniques for Enhanced Vitality

Building upon the foundational practices of visualization and intention-setting, we now ascend to more advanced meditation techniques designed to cultivate profound vitality and enhance your connection to the life force within. These practices are not merely exercises to boost energy; they are pathways to unlocking deeper levels of consciousness and accelerating your journey towards spiritual enlightenment and the immortality of your soul. Remember, the goal is not just physical well-being, but a holistic transformation that integrates mind, body, and spirit into a harmonious symphony of being.

One powerful technique is Trataka, the ancient practice of gazing meditation. This involves focusing your gaze on a single point, typically a candle flame or a visual representation of a deity or symbol that resonates deeply with you. Begin by sitting comfortably in a quiet space, your spine erect but relaxed. Choose your focal point and gently fix your gaze upon it without straining your eyes. Allow your mind to settle, observing the flickering of the flame, the subtle nuances of color and light. As your focus intensifies, you'll notice the mind becoming calmer, thoughts gradually subsiding like ripples in a still pond. Maintain this gaze for a few minutes, gradually increasing the duration as you become more comfortable. When your eyes begin to feel tired, gently close them and continue the meditation internally, visualizing the image you were focusing on. Trataka strengthens your concentration, improves eyesight, and deepens your connection to your inner stillness, preparing the ground for higher states of awareness.

The benefits of Trataka extend beyond improved focus. By consistently practicing this technique, you strengthen your mental fortitude, develop unwavering attention, and foster inner clarity. The focused gaze helps to calm the nervous system, reducing stress and anxiety while promoting a sense of deep tranquility. Regular practice can even enhance your intuition, allowing you to perceive subtle energies and insights more clearly. Remember, consistency is key; even short daily sessions can yield significant results over time. Start with shorter durations and gradually increase the time as your comfort level grows. Listen to your body and cease the practice if you experience any discomfort.

Another advanced technique to enhance vitality is chakra balancing meditation. Our seven primary chakras are energy centers along the spine, each associated with specific aspects of our physical, emotional, and spiritual well-being. When these chakras are balanced and flowing freely, we experience a state of vibrant health, harmony, and inner peace. Imbalanced chakras, on the other hand, can manifest as physical ailments, emotional disturbances, or spiritual stagnation.

To balance your chakras, begin by finding a quiet and comfortable space. Assume a meditative posture, either sitting or lying down. Close your eyes and bring your awareness to your breath. Visualize each chakra in turn, starting with the root chakra at the base of your spine, then moving up through the sacral, solar plexus, heart, throat, third eye, and crown chakras. For each chakra, visualize its associated color (red for root, orange for sacral, etc.) and imagine a radiant light filling the chakra, clearing any blockages or imbalances. You might also use affirmations or mantras associated with each chakra to amplify the healing energy. For example, for the root chakra, you could repeat affirmations like "I am grounded, safe, and secure." For the heart chakra, you might use affirmations like "I am open to love and compassion."

While visualizing, pay attention to any sensations or emotions that arise. These are important clues to areas needing attention. If you feel a blockage or heaviness in a particular chakra, focus your attention and energy on that area, visualizing it clearing and opening. Chakra balancing meditations require consistent practice to yield significant results. Regular practice, even for short periods, can lead to increased energy levels, emotional stability, and improved physical health. Remember, the intention is to bring balance and harmony to your entire energy system.

Beyond Trataka and chakra balancing, explore other advanced practices such as pranayama (yogic breathing techniques), Kundalini awakening meditations (under the guidance of an experienced instructor), and sound healing meditations using singing bowls or other instruments. These practices can further enhance your vitality, deepen your spiritual connection, and accelerate your progress toward spiritual enlightenment. However, it's crucial to approach these advanced practices with caution and respect. Some, especially those involving Kundalini awakening, should only be undertaken under the guidance of a qualified and experienced instructor to prevent potential adverse effects.

Remember, the path to spiritual enlightenment is a journey of self-discovery, patience, and consistent effort. These advanced techniques offer powerful tools to enhance your journey, but their effectiveness depends on your dedication, commitment, and willingness to delve deep within yourself. Approach these practices with reverence, respect, and awareness of your own limitations. Always listen to your body and cease any practice if you experience discomfort or overwhelming sensations.

Furthermore, it's important to address the importance of integrating these advanced meditation practices into your daily life. The benefits of these techniques are not limited to the time spent meditating; they extend into every aspect of your life, enriching your interactions, enhancing your creativity, and improving your overall well-being. By cultivating inner peace and harmony through regular meditation, you can navigate life's challenges with greater ease, resilience, and clarity.

The enhanced vitality you cultivate through advanced meditation practices will manifest not only in your physical energy levels but also in your mental clarity, emotional stability, and spiritual depth. It's a holistic transformation, encompassing all aspects of your being. This vitality is not merely a fleeting energy boost; it's a sustainable and deep-seated well-being that empowers you to live a more fulfilling and meaningful life. It nourishes the soul, allowing it to thrive and flourish.

As you progress, you may find that these practices become integrated into your daily life, seamlessly blending into your routine. The calm focus and inner awareness cultivated through meditation become tools you use not just during your dedicated practice but also throughout your day. You might find yourself responding to stressful situations with greater calmness and equanimity, or perhaps finding creative solutions to problems more readily. This is the true power of advanced meditation: it's not merely an isolated practice, but a way of life.

The ultimate goal of these practices is to connect you more deeply with your true self, your essence, the immortal soul within. By cultivating inner peace, balance, and vitality, you are not simply extending your physical lifespan; you are extending the vibrancy and richness of your spiritual life. This is the path to the immortality of the soul – not a literal immortality in the physical sense, but a transcendence beyond the limitations of the physical body, a connection to something larger, more profound, and eternally enduring.

Throughout this journey, it's crucial to maintain a balanced approach. While embracing these advanced techniques, remember the importance of self-care, proper nutrition, and sufficient rest. These practices are meant to enhance your well-being, not to exhaust or deplete you. Listen to your body's signals, and don't push yourself beyond your limits. Progressive deepening of practice, with mindful attention to your physical and emotional well-being, is the key to sustainable results.

Finally, remember the power of community. Sharing your experiences with others who are on a similar path can be immensely supportive. Consider joining a meditation group or finding a mentor who can offer guidance and support as you delve into these deeper practices. The journey towards spiritual enlightenment is often richer and more rewarding when shared with others. The collective energy and mutual support can amplify your own progress and deepen your understanding of these profound techniques. Remember, you are not alone on this path.

Overcoming Obstacles and Challenges on the Path

The path to unlocking your inner potential through meditation, while profoundly rewarding, is rarely a smooth, uninterrupted journey. Like scaling a majestic mountain, you'll encounter challenging terrain, unexpected weather shifts, and moments of doubt that test your resolve. Yet, it is within these very challenges that the true strength and resilience of the spirit are revealed.

One of the most common obstacles encountered during meditation is restlessness. The mind, accustomed to a constant stream of thoughts and sensations, initially resists the stillness and quietude of meditative practice. It fidgets, seeking distraction in the form of external stimuli or internal ruminations. You might find yourself constantly shifting positions, your mind racing with to-do lists, worries about the future, or regrets about the past. This restlessness is perfectly normal; it's the mind's natural resistance to change. The key is not to fight this resistance but to acknowledge it with compassionate awareness.

To counter restlessness, begin by focusing intently on your breath. Notice the gentle rise and fall of your abdomen, the subtle coolness of the air entering your nostrils, and the warmth of the air leaving. When your mind wanders – and it inevitably will – simply acknowledge the thought or sensation without judgment, gently redirecting your attention back to your breath. Think of it like guiding a playful puppy back to its leash; it might pull and tug, but with gentle persistence, you can bring it back to focus.

Another prevalent challenge is distractions. External sounds, sensations, and even subtle internal bodily discomforts can interrupt your meditative state. These distractions, while irritating, are valuable opportunities to cultivate your capacity for focus and concentration. Instead of becoming frustrated or abandoning your practice, practice observing these distractions with a detached curiosity. Acknowledge their presence, notice them without judgment, and then gently shift your attention back to your chosen focus – your breath, a mantra, or a visualization.

Negative thoughts, too, often arise during meditation. Doubt, self-criticism, and feelings of inadequacy can surface, threatening to derail your practice. These negative thoughts are often deeply ingrained patterns of thinking, habits of mind that have been cultivated over years, even decades. Recognizing these patterns is the first step in overcoming them. When negative thoughts appear, don't try to suppress them; rather, acknowledge them with gentle acceptance, recognizing them as temporary visitors to your mind, not reflections of your inherent worth.

Imagine these thoughts as clouds drifting across the vast expanse of the sky. They may temporarily obscure the sun, but they do not diminish its power. Similarly, negative thoughts may momentarily cloud your peace, but they do not diminish your inner strength and capacity for serenity. Allow these thoughts to pass through your awareness, observing them without judgment, like watching the clouds drift by.

Maintaining consistency in meditation is crucial for experiencing its transformative power. However, life inevitably throws curveballs: unexpected commitments, illness, or emotional turmoil can disrupt your practice. When faced with such setbacks, don't beat yourself up. Instead, approach these interruptions with self-compassion and understanding. Remember that your meditation practice is a marathon, not a sprint. Even a few minutes of mindful breathing each day can make a profound difference. Be kind to yourself, acknowledge any challenges you've faced, and gently resume your practice when you're able.

Creating a supportive environment for your meditation is also essential. Find a quiet space where you can sit or lie down comfortably, free from interruptions. Consider using calming music or nature sounds to create a soothing ambiance. If you're finding it difficult to quiet your mind, try meditating with a guided meditation app. These apps can provide structure and support, guiding you through various techniques and helping you develop a consistent practice.

Furthermore, engage in self-care practices to support your meditation. Regular exercise, healthy eating, and sufficient sleep are crucial for maintaining both physical and mental well-being. These practices will not only enhance the quality of your meditation but also increase your overall resilience and capacity for coping with life's challenges. Remember, meditation is not simply a practice; it's a lifestyle, a journey of self-discovery and self-acceptance.

Another aspect of overcoming obstacles is to remember that setbacks are not failures, but rather valuable opportunities for growth and learning. Every time you encounter a challenge, you gain a deeper understanding of your own mind, your strengths, and your limitations. You learn to cultivate patience, compassion, and resilience – qualities that are essential not only for your meditation practice but for navigating life's complexities as well.

Consider journaling your experiences. This can provide a valuable tool for reflecting on your progress, identifying recurring challenges, and celebrating your achievements. Writing down your thoughts and feelings can help you process any emotional blockages that may be impeding your spiritual progress.

The journey of meditation, much like life itself, is one of continuous learning and growth. There will be days of profound clarity and moments of frustrating struggle. Embrace both with equal acceptance and understanding. Remember that the path to unlocking your inner potential is a personal one; there is no right or wrong way to meditate. The most important thing is to maintain a consistent and compassionate approach to your practice.

Through diligent practice and a compassionate approach, you will gradually cultivate greater mental clarity, emotional stability, and an unwavering sense of inner peace. The challenges you encounter along the way are not roadblocks, but stepping stones on the path to unlocking your deepest potential and experiencing the transformative power of meditation. Embrace the journey, be patient with yourself, and celebrate every small victory along the way. The rewards of a consistent meditation practice are immeasurable, leading to a richer, more fulfilling, and profoundly meaningful life. It is a journey of self-discovery, a pathway to unlocking your inherent potential and connecting with the boundless source of life force within you. The perseverance you demonstrate in facing and overcoming obstacles will ultimately strengthen your spirit and deepen your connection to the divine essence that resides within each of us. The path may be challenging, but the destination is worth the effort.

Cultivating SelfCompassion and SelfAcceptance

The journey inward, towards unlocking your inner potential through meditation, is inextricably linked to cultivating a profound sense of self-compassion and self-acceptance. Without this inner harmony, the transformative power of meditation can be significantly diminished. We often treat ourselves with far less kindness and understanding than we would offer a dear friend struggling with similar challenges. This inner critic, constantly judging and berating, creates a barrier to our spiritual growth and prevents us from fully embracing the peace and tranquility that meditation offers.

To truly unlock your inner potential, you must first cultivate a loving relationship with yourself, a relationship built on understanding, forgiveness, and unwavering acceptance. This involves confronting the deeply ingrained patterns of self-criticism that may have developed over years, perhaps even decades. These patterns, often rooted in childhood experiences or societal conditioning, can subtly sabotage our efforts to achieve inner peace and self-realization. They whisper doubts, magnify flaws, and prevent us from celebrating our achievements, big or small.

One powerful technique for releasing self-criticism is mindful self-awareness. This involves paying close attention to your inner dialogue, observing your thoughts and feelings without judgment. Notice the critical voice, the harsh self-assessment, the negative self-talk. Simply observe it, without engaging with it. Imagine it as a cloud drifting across the sky —watch it pass, acknowledge its presence, but don't let it dictate your mood or actions. This practice of detached observation helps to create a space between you and your critical thoughts, gradually weakening their hold over you.

Another powerful tool is the practice of self-compassion meditation. This involves focusing on your breath and gently bringing your attention to any feelings of self-criticism or self-judgment. As these feelings arise, imagine extending a warm embrace to yourself, offering words of comfort and understanding. You might say silently, "It's okay, I'm doing my best," or "I forgive myself for my imperfections." This act of self-nurturing, of offering kindness and compassion to your inner self, is profoundly transformative. It begins to dissolve the armor of self-criticism, replacing it with a sense of acceptance and self-love.

Self-forgiveness is a crucial element in this process. We all make mistakes, experience setbacks, and engage in actions that we later regret. Holding onto these past transgressions, replaying them in our minds, only perpetuates feelings of guilt and shame. Self-forgiveness is not about condoning harmful behavior; it's about recognizing our inherent fallibility, learning from our mistakes, and choosing to move forward with compassion and understanding. Imagine yourself as a compassionate friend witnessing your past mistakes. What would you say to that friend? Extend that same level of kindness and understanding to yourself. The journey towards self-forgiveness is often gradual, but the rewards are immeasurable.

Overcoming limiting beliefs is another essential step in cultivating self-acceptance. These are the deeply held negative beliefs about ourselves that dictate our behavior and limit our potential. Beliefs such as "I'm not good enough," "I'm not worthy of love," or "I'll never succeed," can become self-fulfilling prophecies. Through meditation and self-reflection, you can identify and challenge these limiting beliefs. Ask yourself: Is this belief truly accurate? What evidence supports it, and what evidence contradicts it? By questioning these beliefs and consciously replacing them with more positive and empowering affirmations, you can gradually transform your self-perception and unlock your true potential. Affirmations such as "I am worthy of love and happiness," "I am capable of achieving my goals," and "I am strong and resilient," can be profoundly effective in reshaping your self-image.

The integration of self-compassion and self-acceptance into your meditation practice is not a passive endeavor; it requires consistent effort and conscious intention. It involves incorporating elements such as mindful self-awareness, self-compassion meditation, and self-forgiveness into your daily routine. Begin by setting aside a few minutes each day to practice these techniques. As you become more comfortable, gradually increase the duration of your practice.

Consider using guided meditations specifically designed to cultivate self-compassion. Many such meditations are readily available online or through meditation apps. These guided sessions can provide a supportive framework for exploring your emotions, releasing self-criticism, and fostering a sense of self-love. Additionally, journaling can be a valuable tool. Write down your thoughts and feelings, both positive and negative. Exploring your inner world through writing can provide insights into your limiting beliefs and help you identify areas where you need to cultivate more self-compassion.

Remember, the process of cultivating self-compassion and self-acceptance is a journey, not a destination. There will be times when you falter, when self-criticism resurfaces, and when you feel discouraged. This is entirely normal. Be patient with yourself, acknowledge your imperfections, and continue to practice self-compassion with unwavering commitment. Each small step forward, each act of self-kindness, contributes to the overall transformation.

The benefits of integrating self-compassion and self-acceptance into your meditation practice extend far beyond simply feeling better about yourself. As you cultivate inner peace and harmony, you will experience a greater sense of resilience in the face of life's challenges. You will find it easier to manage stress, navigate difficult emotions, and maintain a sense of balance amidst chaos. Your relationships with others will deepen as you approach them with the same compassion and understanding that you extend to yourself. Your creativity and productivity will flourish as you release the burden of self-doubt and embrace your true potential. Ultimately, the cultivation of self-compassion and self-acceptance is not merely a spiritual practice, but a foundation for a richer, more fulfilling, and profoundly meaningful life. It is a vital component of the journey towards unlocking your inner potential and experiencing the transformative power of meditation, leading you closer to the immortality of your soul, not merely in a spiritual sense, but in the lasting impact you have on the world and the legacy you leave behind. This inner peace and self-acceptance ripple outwards, affecting everyone you encounter and creating a more compassionate and harmonious world. The journey is personal, but the impact is universal. Embrace the process, for it is in this journey of self-discovery that true transformation lies. And remember, even in the midst of challenges, the unwavering presence of self-compassion is your constant companion, guiding you along the path towards inner peace and ultimately, towards the boundless potential within.

Developing Intuition and Inner Wisdom

Building upon the foundation of self-compassion and self-acceptance established in our journey inward, we now embark on a deeper exploration of the transformative power of meditation: the cultivation of intuition and inner wisdom. This innate capacity to access deeper knowledge and understanding, often beyond the realm of conscious thought, lies dormant within each of us, waiting to be awakened. Meditation provides the fertile ground for this awakening, nurturing the quiet space where the whispers of intuition can be heard above the clamor of the everyday world.

The process begins with a fundamental shift in perspective. We must move beyond the reliance on purely rational, analytical thinking and embrace a more holistic approach, recognizing the intuitive realm as a valid and crucial source of guidance. This isn't about dismissing logic or intellect; rather, it's about integrating intuition as a complementary and often more insightful form of knowing. Imagine it as two wings of a bird—logic and intuition—working together to allow for graceful flight. One without the other leads to a limited and less effective journey.

One of the most effective techniques for developing intuition through meditation involves focusing on the breath. As we discussed in the previous chapter, controlling our breath is a fundamental aspect of meditative practice. However, here, we focus not merely on the mechanics, but on the subtle sensations associated with the breath. Notice the coolness of the air as it enters your nostrils, the warmth as it leaves. Feel the gentle rise and fall of your chest or abdomen. This focused attention quiets the mental chatter, creating a space for the subtle whispers of intuition to emerge. These whispers may present themselves as fleeting images, feelings, or gut sensations – a sudden sense of knowing, often difficult to articulate logically, yet undeniably compelling.

As you deepen your meditative practice, you'll become more attuned to these subtle cues. It's like learning a new language; at first, you may struggle to decipher the meaning, but with consistent practice, you will develop fluency. Begin by setting a specific intention for your meditation. Perhaps you're facing a difficult decision, or you're seeking clarity on a particular issue. As you focus on your breath, gently allow your mind to wander towards the question at hand, observing your thoughts and feelings without judgment. Pay close attention to any recurring images, symbols, or emotions that arise. These often hold the key to your intuitive understanding.

Journaling can be a powerful tool in this process. After each meditation session, take a few moments to record your experience. Note any insights, images, or feelings that arose during your practice. Don't censor yourself; simply allow the words to flow onto the page. Over time, you'll begin to recognize patterns and themes, gaining a deeper understanding of your intuitive guidance system. These seemingly random thoughts and feelings often point towards a larger truth, often a truth that logic alone cannot uncover.

Let's consider an example. Imagine you're contemplating a career change. You've meticulously weighed the pros and cons of each option, analyzed market trends, and consulted with mentors. Yet, you still feel a sense of uncertainty. Through meditation, you might find yourself repeatedly drawn to images of nature, or perhaps a recurring feeling of calm and freedom associated with a particular field. This seemingly unrelated imagery might point towards a career path that aligns more deeply with your inner self, offering a level of fulfillment beyond what a purely rational analysis can reveal. Your intuition may not provide concrete answers, but it offers a compass to guide you towards a path of greater alignment and purpose.

Another crucial element in developing your intuition is to cultivate a sense of inner stillness. This is achieved not through forceful suppression of thoughts, but through gentle observation. When thoughts arise, acknowledge them without judgment, allowing them to pass like clouds across the sky. The goal is not to eliminate thoughts entirely—that is impossible—but to create a space of quiet awareness where the subtle voice of intuition can be heard. This stillness allows for a clear connection to your inner wisdom, a connection often obscured by the relentless activity of the conscious mind.

It's vital to distinguish between true intuition and ego-driven thoughts. Ego-driven thoughts often present themselves as strong opinions or judgments, fueled by fear, insecurity, or a desire for validation. Intuition, on the other hand, tends to be more subtle, peaceful, and aligned with your overall well-being. It may offer gentle guidance, a sense of knowing without needing to forcefully convince or justify itself. Developing this discernment takes time and practice. It requires a willingness to question your own thoughts and feelings, to examine their origin and their impact on your overall sense of peace.

Over time, with consistent meditation practice and focused attention on the subtle cues of your intuition, you'll develop a greater capacity to trust your inner wisdom. This trust will empower you to make decisions aligned with your deepest values and aspirations, leading to a more fulfilling and meaningful life. Remember, the development of intuition is not a linear process. There will be moments of clarity and moments of confusion. Embrace both as part of the journey. The key is consistent practice, self-compassion, and a willingness to listen to the quiet voice within.

As we move further along this path, we discover that intuition is not merely a source of guidance for personal decisions; it also plays a significant role in connecting us with something larger than ourselves, a sense of the divine, or a universal consciousness. As our capacity for inner stillness increases through consistent meditation, we become more attuned to subtle energies, synchronicities, and seemingly miraculous occurrences that confirm our connection to this greater reality. These experiences often defy logical explanation, yet they resonate deeply within our being, strengthening our belief in the power of intuition and its connection to a profound spiritual reality.

Intuition is not a magical ability bestowed upon a select few; it is an innate capacity that resides within each of us. Through the practice of meditation, we cultivate the stillness and awareness necessary to access this inner wisdom, transforming our lives from a reactive to a responsive state. By tuning into the subtle whispers of intuition, we create a life that is not merely lived, but consciously created and directed. It is a life infused with purpose, meaning, and a profound connection to our inner self and the larger universe around us.

Moreover, the cultivation of intuition enhances our capacity for empathy and compassion. As we become more attuned to our own inner landscape, we develop a deeper understanding of the experiences of others. We begin to sense their emotions, understand their motivations, and respond with greater kindness and understanding. This heightened sensitivity fosters stronger relationships, enhances communication, and ultimately contributes to a more harmonious and compassionate world.

In practical terms, consider the everyday decisions we face. Should you accept a new job offer? Should you move to a new city? Should you invest in a particular venture? While rational analysis plays a role, often intuition provides the final, decisive nudge. That feeling of deep resonance, the sense of "knowing" that transcends logical reasoning—this is the voice of your intuition guiding you towards a path aligned with your highest good.

Let's delve deeper into how intuition manifests in different aspects of our lives. In our relationships, intuition often alerts us to hidden dynamics or unspoken tensions. It might be a gut feeling telling you that something is not quite right in a certain interaction or partnership. This feeling is not necessarily based on concrete evidence, but rather on a deeper, intuitive understanding of the emotional undercurrents. Paying attention to these signals can help us navigate relationships with greater awareness and sensitivity.

In our professional lives, intuition can be a powerful asset in decision-making. A seasoned entrepreneur might sense a market opportunity before the data supports it or recognize a potential problem before it becomes a crisis. This intuitive insight, coupled with rational analysis, enables them to make informed decisions and stay ahead of the curve. In creative endeavors, intuition is even more indispensable. Artists, writers, and musicians often rely on their intuition to guide their creative process, allowing them to access inspiration and generate innovative ideas beyond the reach of conscious thought.

The journey of developing intuition and inner wisdom is a lifelong endeavor. It is a continuous process of refinement, deepening, and integration. It requires patience, self-compassion, and a willingness to embrace the unknown. Yet, the rewards are immeasurable. As we cultivate this inner capacity, we step into a greater realm of self-awareness, unlocking our true potential and living a life of greater purpose, fulfillment, and deep connection to the divine. This is the path to true immortality of the soul—not in a literal sense, but in the enduring impact we have on the world and the legacy of love, wisdom, and compassion that we leave behind. This legacy extends far beyond our physical existence, echoing in the hearts and minds of those we touch. It is a testament to the power of a life lived authentically, guided by the intuitive wisdom residing within us.

The Role of Gratitude and Appreciation in Spiritual Growth

Having cultivated a deeper connection to our intuition and inner wisdom through meditation, we now turn our attention to another powerful tool for spiritual growth: gratitude. Gratitude isn't merely a pleasant emotion; it's a transformative force that can reshape our perception of reality, profoundly impacting our well-being and accelerating our spiritual journey. It acts as a bridge, connecting us to the abundance that already surrounds us, even amidst challenges. It shifts our focus from what we lack to what we possess, fostering a sense of contentment and appreciation that nourishes the soul.

The practice of gratitude isn't about ignoring hardship or pretending that everything is perfect. Instead, it's about acknowledging the good amidst the bad, recognizing the blessings both large and small that enrich our lives. This involves consciously shifting our awareness from a state of deficiency to one of abundance, actively seeking and celebrating the positive aspects of our experience. This conscious shift is where the true power of gratitude lies—not passively noticing good things, but actively seeking them out and acknowledging their presence in our lives. It's a deliberate choice, a conscious act of appreciation that transforms our internal landscape.

Consider this: when we focus on what we lack, we fuel feelings of discontent, frustration, and even resentment. This negativity creates a vibrational mismatch with the universal energy of abundance, hindering our ability to attract positive experiences. Gratitude, on the other hand, acts as a magnet, drawing more positive energy into our lives. It raises our vibrational frequency, aligning us with the flow of abundance and attracting more opportunities for growth and fulfillment.

Many people mistakenly associate gratitude with passive acceptance, believing it means we must be content with any circumstance, regardless of its challenges. This is a misconception. Gratitude doesn't necessitate blind acceptance of difficult situations; rather, it's about finding the silver lining, recognizing the lessons learned, and appreciating the resilience we discover within ourselves as we navigate life's complexities. It allows us to find meaning and purpose even in difficult times, knowing that challenges often pave the way for personal growth and spiritual evolution.

For example, consider a period of unemployment. While the experience is undoubtedly stressful, gratitude practice invites us to acknowledge the extra time it may provide for self-reflection, personal development, or pursuing long-deferred passions. It allows us to appreciate the support of loved ones, the lessons learned about resilience, and the opportunity to re-evaluate our career path. Similarly, a difficult relationship, though painful, may lead us to understand our own needs and boundaries better, providing a springboard for future, healthier connections.

The practice of gratitude can manifest in various ways. A simple yet powerful method is to maintain a gratitude journal. Each day, take a few minutes to write down three things you are grateful for. These can be anything, from the warmth of the sun on your skin to a meaningful conversation with a loved one, a successful project at work, or simply a quiet moment of peace. The key is to focus on the specifics —rather than simply writing "I'm grateful for my health," delve into the details: "I'm grateful for the energy I have today that allowed me to take a long walk in nature." This level of detail amplifies the impact of the exercise, deepening your appreciation and fostering a stronger sense of gratitude.

Another powerful technique is to incorporate gratitude into your daily meditation practice. After finding a comfortable seated position and settling into a state of quiet awareness, take a few moments to reflect on the aspects of your life that bring you joy, contentment, and peace. Focus on the feeling of gratitude arising within you, allowing it to permeate your being. Visualize the positive energy flowing through your body, expanding outwards to encompass all aspects of your life. This practice not only cultivates a deeper sense of appreciation but also enhances your meditative experience, deepening your connection to your inner self and the divine.

Furthermore, expressing gratitude verbally is a powerful way to amplify its effects. Take the time to express your appreciation to those who have positively impacted your life. A simple "thank you" can go a long way, fostering stronger bonds and creating a ripple effect of positivity. Expressing gratitude can be as simple as a handwritten note, a phone call, or even a heartfelt conversation. The act of expressing your gratitude strengthens your connections with others and reinforces the positive emotions within you.

Beyond individual practice, extending gratitude to the universe or a higher power is equally significant. This practice cultivates a sense of humility and deepens our connection to something larger than ourselves. It allows us to recognize the interconnectedness of all things and appreciate the abundance that sustains our lives. This perspective shift allows us to view challenges not as isolated events but as part of a larger, unfolding plan, fostering acceptance and peace of mind.

Incorporating gratitude into our daily lives isn't about forcing positivity; it's about cultivating a mindful appreciation for the present moment. It's about consciously choosing to focus on the positive aspects of our experiences, however small they may seem. This conscious choice, this deliberate act of appreciation, is what transforms our perception of reality and opens the door to a more fulfilling and meaningful life.

It's crucial to understand that gratitude is not a quick fix for solving all life's problems. It's a continuous practice, a lifelong journey of cultivating a heart of appreciation. Some days, it may feel easier than others. There will be times when challenges seem overwhelming, and finding gratitude may feel difficult. However, it's precisely during these times that the practice of gratitude is most essential. It's through these challenges that we discover our strength, resilience, and capacity for growth. Holding onto gratitude, even when faced with adversity, helps us to maintain a positive outlook and strengthens our connection to the divine.

Furthermore, the act of appreciating the small things—a beautiful sunset, a warm cup of tea, the laughter of a child— can be remarkably powerful. These simple pleasures, often overlooked in the rush of daily life, can be potent reminders of the abundance that surrounds us. By actively seeking and appreciating these moments of joy, we cultivate a deeper sense of contentment and satisfaction, nourishing our souls and enriching our lives.

The integration of gratitude into our meditation practice enhances its transformative power. The meditative state allows us to quiet the mind's chatter, creating space for appreciation to blossom. As we focus on the breath, we become more present, more aware of the subtle joys and wonders that often escape our notice in the everyday hustle and bustle. This deeper level of presence allows us to fully appreciate the richness and beauty of our experiences, enhancing the transformative power of gratitude.

Finally, remember that gratitude is a reciprocal energy. When we express gratitude, we not only benefit ourselves, but we also inspire gratitude in others. This ripple effect of positivity creates a harmonious environment, fostering connection and promoting well-being. By actively cultivating gratitude, we not only transform our own lives, but we also contribute to creating a more loving and compassionate world. The practice of gratitude is not simply a spiritual exercise; it's a path to a more fulfilling and meaningful existence, a path that leads us towards the immortality of the soul – not in the literal sense, but in the enduring legacy of love, appreciation, and compassion that we leave behind. It's a testament to a life lived with a heart filled with thankfulness, a life deeply connected to the divine, a life that echoes long after our physical presence is gone. This enduring legacy is the true essence of spiritual immortality.

Achieving Peak Performance Through Mindfulness

Building upon the foundation of gratitude and inner wisdom cultivated through meditation, we now explore how this practice directly translates into achieving peak performance in our daily lives. The seemingly disparate worlds of spiritual growth and worldly success are, in reality, deeply intertwined. Meditation, far from being a passive retreat from the demands of life, is a powerful tool for sharpening our minds, enhancing our emotional resilience, and ultimately, propelling us toward our goals. It's a path to unlocking our innate potential, allowing us to operate at a higher level of efficiency and effectiveness.

The key lies in cultivating mindfulness – a state of present moment awareness – through consistent meditation practice. Mindfulness isn't just about sitting quietly; it's about bringing this awareness into every aspect of our lives. It's about observing our thoughts, emotions, and sensations without judgment, allowing us to respond to situations rather than react impulsively. This heightened awareness is the cornerstone of peak performance.

In the workplace, for instance, mindfulness translates into increased productivity and creativity. When we approach our tasks with a clear, focused mind, free from the distractions of worry or anxiety, our ability to concentrate improves dramatically. We become more efficient, making fewer mistakes and completing our work more effectively. Moreover, mindfulness fosters creativity by allowing us to approach challenges with a fresh perspective, unburdened by ingrained thought patterns or habitual responses. We become more open to innovative solutions, recognizing opportunities that might otherwise be missed.

Consider the experience of a surgeon performing a complex operation. The surgeon's ability to remain calm, focused, and present in the moment is paramount to success. Years of training and skill are undoubtedly essential, but the mental state cultivated through mindfulness meditation significantly enhances their ability to execute the procedure with precision and grace, minimizing risk and maximizing positive outcomes. This same principle applies to any profession, from a software engineer meticulously debugging code to a teacher engaging students in a dynamic learning environment.

Similarly, mindfulness profoundly impacts our interpersonal relationships. When we approach our interactions with others from a place of present moment awareness, we are better able to listen deeply, empathize genuinely, and communicate effectively. We are less likely to misinterpret others' intentions or react defensively to perceived slights. Instead, we respond with compassion and understanding, fostering stronger, more meaningful connections.

Imagine a conflict arising between colleagues at work. In the absence of mindfulness, the situation might escalate into a heated argument, damaging relationships and hindering productivity. However, if both parties approach the situation with mindful awareness, they are more likely to listen to each other's perspectives with empathy, identify the root cause of the conflict, and collaboratively find a mutually agreeable solution. This transformation from conflict to collaboration is a direct result of the emotional regulation and clear-headedness cultivated through meditation.

The benefits of mindfulness extend beyond the professional and interpersonal spheres. It impacts our overall well-being, reducing stress, anxiety, and depression. By regularly engaging in meditation, we train our minds to observe our emotions without getting carried away by them. When challenging thoughts or feelings arise, we are less likely to be overwhelmed, able instead to respond with greater composure and resilience. This emotional regulation has a ripple effect, positively impacting our physical health as well. Reduced stress levels contribute to improved cardiovascular health, better sleep quality, and a strengthened immune system.

Furthermore, mindfulness allows us to cultivate a deeper appreciation for the present moment. We become less preoccupied with the past or anxious about the future, learning to find joy and contentment in the here and now. This shift in perspective can be profoundly transformative, leading to a greater sense of peace and fulfillment in our lives. The seemingly mundane aspects of daily life—the taste of our morning coffee, the warmth of the sun on our skin, the laughter of a loved one—become opportunities for profound appreciation, enriching our experiences and enhancing our overall sense of well-being. This heightened appreciation for the present moment is intrinsically linked to the concept of spiritual immortality, as it allows us to fully inhabit and savor the preciousness of each moment.

The path to achieving peak performance through mindfulness isn't a quick fix or a shortcut to success. It requires consistent effort and dedication. Just as a musician practices scales and exercises to refine their technique, we must consistently engage in meditation to cultivate the mental and emotional clarity necessary for peak performance. The benefits, however, are immeasurable. It's not just about achieving greater productivity or success in our worldly endeavors; it's about living a more fulfilling, meaningful, and ultimately more joyful life.

Consider the impact of mindfulness on physical athletes. Top performers in sports such as golf, tennis, or archery often incorporate mindfulness techniques into their training regimens. The ability to focus intently on the present moment, to block out distractions, and to remain calm under pressure is crucial for optimal performance. Mindfulness allows athletes to refine their skills, improve their consistency, and achieve peak performance in high-stakes situations. The same principle applies to artists, musicians, writers, and anyone striving for excellence in their chosen field. The clarity and focus cultivated through meditation provide a competitive edge, allowing individuals to excel in their chosen pursuit.

In addition to its impact on performance, mindfulness plays a vital role in managing stress, a common obstacle to productivity and well-being. Stress can manifest in various ways – physical symptoms like headaches or digestive issues, emotional symptoms like irritability or anxiety, and cognitive symptoms like difficulty concentrating or making decisions. Mindfulness meditation provides a powerful antidote to stress by helping us regulate our nervous system response to stressors. Instead of reacting impulsively to stressful situations, we learn to observe our reactions without judgment, creating space between the stimulus and our response. This creates a sense of calm and control, reducing the negative impact of stress on our physical and mental health. As a result, we are better equipped to handle challenges, both big and small.

The practice of mindfulness is not merely a technique to be mastered; it's a journey of self-discovery. As we cultivate greater awareness of our thoughts and emotions, we gain a deeper understanding of ourselves, our strengths, and our weaknesses. This self-awareness is essential for personal growth and development. It allows us to identify areas where we need to improve, to set realistic goals, and to develop strategies for achieving them. This process of self-reflection, guided by the stillness of meditation, allows us to align our actions with our values, leading to a more authentic and purposeful life.

Finally, the connection between mindfulness, peak performance, and spiritual growth is profound. By cultivating inner peace and clarity through meditation, we tap into a deeper wellspring of creativity, resilience, and compassion. This transformative process extends beyond the boundaries of personal achievement, impacting our relationships with others and our contribution to the world. It is through this integration of worldly success with spiritual depth that we truly unlock our inner potential, experiencing a life of both purpose and fulfillment. This holistic approach to well-being, nurtured through the consistent practice of mindfulness meditation, is the path to not only peak performance but to a life lived with intention, compassion, and a profound connection to something larger than ourselves—a life that resonates with the enduring legacy of the immortal soul.

The Impact of Meditation on the Nervous System

The intricate network of our nervous system, the command center of our being, is profoundly impacted by the practice of meditation. This isn't merely anecdotal; a growing body of scientific research illuminates the profound and measurable changes meditation induces within this complex system. One of the most significant impacts is the reduction of stress, a pervasive modern ailment that wreaks havoc on our physical and mental health. Chronic stress activates the sympathetic nervous system, initiating the "fight-or-flight" response. This involves the release of stress hormones like cortisol and adrenaline, leading to elevated heart rate, blood pressure, and muscle tension. Over time, this constant state of hyper-arousal can damage various systems in the body, contributing to conditions like anxiety, depression, cardiovascular disease, and a weakened immune system.

Meditation, however, offers a powerful antidote. Studies using techniques like fMRI (functional magnetic resonance imaging) have shown that regular meditation practice leads to a decrease in activity in the amygdala, the brain region associated with fear and stress responses. Simultaneously, there's an increase in activity in the prefrontal cortex, the region responsible for executive functions like attention, self-regulation, and emotional control. This shift in brain activity helps to dampen the stress response, allowing the parasympathetic nervous system – responsible for the "rest-and-digest" response – to take over. The result is a state of calm, reduced physiological arousal, and a greater capacity to manage stressful situations.

This physiological shift translates into measurable improvements in several key areas. Sleep, often disrupted by stress and anxiety, is significantly enhanced through regular meditation. Studies have shown that individuals who practice meditation regularly experience deeper, more restorative sleep, leading to improved mood, increased energy levels, and enhanced cognitive function. The restorative nature of sleep allows the body to repair and rejuvenate, contributing to overall well-being and longevity. The improved sleep quality is directly linked to the regulation of the nervous system and its impact on the sleep-wake cycle.

Beyond sleep, meditation demonstrably improves cognitive function. Studies have shown improvements in attention span, working memory, and executive function in individuals who practice meditation regularly. This is likely due to the increased activity in the prefrontal cortex, the brain region responsible for these cognitive processes. The ability to focus attention and resist distractions, key components of meditation practice, directly translate to improved cognitive performance in daily life. This enhanced cognitive function is not only beneficial for daily tasks but also plays a crucial role in maintaining cognitive health as we age, potentially delaying the onset of age-related cognitive decline.

Furthermore, research indicates that meditation can positively influence neuroplasticity – the brain's ability to reorganize itself by forming new neural connections throughout life. This means that through consistent practice, meditation can actually change the physical structure and function of the brain, leading to lasting improvements in mood, behavior, and cognitive function. This neuroplasticity contributes to the overall resilience of the nervous system, enabling it to adapt and cope better with stress and challenges. The brain's ability to adapt and rewire itself is a powerful tool in promoting long-term health and well-being.

The impact extends beyond the brain. Meditation's influence on the autonomic nervous system, the involuntary part of the peripheral nervous system that regulates vital functions like heart rate, breathing, and digestion, is noteworthy. Studies have shown that meditation can lower heart rate variability, indicating a more balanced and regulated autonomic nervous system. This regulation contributes to improved cardiovascular health, reduced risk of heart disease, and overall improved physiological well-being. The reduction in heart rate and blood pressure observed in meditators further reinforces the calming and restorative effects of the practice.

The effects on the enteric nervous system, often referred to as the "second brain" located in the gut, are also being explored. Emerging research suggests that meditation may positively influence gut microbiota composition and function, contributing to better digestion and a healthier gut microbiome. The gut-brain axis, the bidirectional communication pathway between the gut and the brain, plays a vital role in overall health and well-being. By positively influencing the gut, meditation may exert beneficial effects on the brain and nervous system through this crucial connection.

Specific meditation techniques demonstrate varying degrees of impact on the nervous system. Mindfulness meditation, focusing on present moment awareness without judgment, has shown remarkable results in reducing stress and improving attention. Loving-kindness meditation, which cultivates feelings of compassion and goodwill, has been linked to increased levels of oxytocin, a hormone associated with social bonding and well-being. Transcendental meditation (TM), a technique involving the repetition of a mantra, has been shown to reduce blood pressure and improve cardiovascular health. Different styles of meditation, therefore, offer diverse approaches to positively influencing the nervous system, catering to individual preferences and needs.

The scientific community continues to unravel the intricate mechanisms through which meditation affects the nervous system. However, the accumulated evidence is compelling. Meditation's impact extends far beyond mere relaxation; it represents a powerful tool for cultivating a healthier, more resilient, and more balanced nervous system, ultimately contributing to improved overall health, well-being, and potentially, longevity. The ongoing research continues to unveil the myriad ways in which this ancient practice shapes our neurological landscape, offering a scientifically validated path towards a more fulfilling and longer life. The consistent practice of meditation, tailored to individual needs and preferences, becomes a potent investment in the long-term health and well-being of one's nervous system. This, in turn, supports the overarching goal of achieving a harmonious balance between mind, body, and spirit – a cornerstone of the journey to spiritual enlightenment and extended life force. By understanding the scientific underpinnings, we can further appreciate the profound benefits of this transformative practice and integrate it effectively into our lives.

Exploring the Link to Longevity

Our journey into the science of meditation and longevity now leads us to a fascinating frontier: the exploration of telomeres and their relationship to the practice of meditation. Telomeres, those protective caps on the ends of our chromosomes, have emerged as key players in the aging process. Think of them as the plastic tips on shoelaces – they prevent fraying and damage. As we age, these telomeres naturally shorten, and this shortening has been linked to a variety of age-related diseases and decreased lifespan. But what if we could influence this natural process? What if we could, in a sense, slow down the shortening of these protective caps?

Emerging research suggests that meditation may hold the key. Studies have shown a correlation between regular meditation practice and longer telomeres. This isn't to say that meditation will magically reverse aging or grant immortality – that's a narrative often oversimplified in popular culture. However, the evidence suggests that meditation may play a significant role in mitigating the effects of cellular aging, leading to a healthier and potentially longer life.

The mechanisms through which meditation impacts telomere length are still being investigated, but several pathways are being explored. One prominent theory centers on the reduction of stress. As previously discussed, chronic stress significantly accelerates telomere shortening. The constant release of stress hormones like cortisol takes a toll on our cellular health, contributing to the erosion of these protective caps. Meditation, with its ability to calm the nervous system and reduce stress hormone levels, may offer a powerful countermeasure to this process. By fostering a state of relaxation and reducing the body's stress response, meditation may help to preserve telomere length, slowing down the cellular clock.

Another potential mechanism involves the impact of meditation on inflammation. Chronic inflammation is a significant contributor to aging and age-related diseases. It's a silent attacker, damaging cells and tissues over time. Meditation has been shown to have anti-inflammatory effects, potentially reducing the inflammatory load on the body and thereby protecting telomeres from further damage. This anti-inflammatory effect is likely mediated through various pathways, including the modulation of the immune system and the reduction of stress-induced inflammation. The intricate interplay between stress, inflammation, and telomere length highlights the multifaceted benefits of a regular meditation practice.

Furthermore, the impact of meditation on telomere length isn't solely due to physiological changes. The mental and emotional benefits of meditation also play a crucial role. Meditation cultivates a sense of inner peace, emotional regulation, and self-awareness – all of which contribute to a healthier mental state. Chronic mental distress, anxiety, and depression are associated with shorter telomeres. By fostering mental resilience and emotional balance, meditation may indirectly protect telomere length. This highlights the synergistic relationship between mind and body, where mental well-being is intricately linked to physical health and longevity.

The research on meditation and telomere length is still evolving, and more large-scale, long-term studies are needed to definitively establish a causal relationship. However, the existing evidence is encouraging and suggests a potential link between regular meditation practice and longer telomere length. This evidence strengthens the case for meditation as a valuable tool for healthy aging, complementing other lifestyle factors such as healthy diet, regular exercise, and sufficient sleep. It's crucial to remember that meditation is not a magical cure-all, but rather a complementary practice that can contribute to a holistic approach to health and well-being.

Let's delve deeper into the specifics of the studies that have explored this fascinating connection. One notable study published in the journal *Psychosomatic Medicine* examined the effects of a mindfulness-based stress reduction (MBSR) program on telomere length in women with metastatic breast cancer. The results showed that participants who completed the MBSR program exhibited significantly less telomere shortening compared to a control group. This suggests that the structured meditation and mindfulness practices inherent in MBSR could have a protective effect on telomere length, even in the face of a serious health challenge.

Another study, published in the journal *Biological Psychiatry* , investigated the relationship between meditation experience and telomere length in a group of healthy individuals. The researchers found a positive correlation between the duration of meditation practice and telomere length. This finding reinforces the idea that consistent and long-term meditation practice may have a cumulative effect on telomere maintenance. While correlation does not equal causation, these findings suggest a compelling potential link that warrants further investigation.

It's important to note that the studies conducted so far have varied in their methodologies, sample sizes, and the types of meditation practices employed. This makes it difficult to draw definitive conclusions. However, the consistent findings across multiple studies hinting at a positive association between meditation and telomere length are encouraging. Further research is needed to clarify the specific mechanisms involved, identify the optimal types of meditation for telomere preservation, and determine the ideal duration and intensity of meditation practice for maximum benefit.

Beyond the specific studies, it's also crucial to consider the broader context of lifestyle factors that influence telomere length. While meditation may offer a significant contribution, it's not a standalone solution. A holistic approach encompassing various lifestyle choices – a balanced diet rich in antioxidants and anti-inflammatory nutrients, regular physical activity, sufficient sleep, stress management techniques beyond meditation, and strong social connections – all play a crucial role in maintaining telomere length and promoting healthy aging. Meditation can be considered a valuable component of this comprehensive strategy, working synergistically with other healthy habits to maximize the impact on cellular health.

The emerging research linking meditation to telomere length offers a glimpse into the profound and far-reaching effects of this ancient practice. It underscores the powerful interconnectedness between our minds, our bodies, and our cellular processes. By fostering inner peace, reducing stress, and modulating inflammation, meditation may contribute significantly to slowing down the cellular aging process. This adds a new dimension to our understanding of the profound benefits of meditation, further cementing its place as a valuable tool for not just spiritual growth but also for improving physical health and extending lifespan.

The pursuit of longevity is not merely about extending our physical lifespan; it's about enhancing the quality of our years. Meditation, in its capacity to impact telomere length, offers a path towards both. By cultivating a state of inner balance and reducing the damaging effects of chronic stress and inflammation, meditation contributes to a healthier, more vibrant life, allowing us to live more fully, experience deeper connection, and engage more meaningfully with the world around us. The journey to spiritual enlightenment, as envisioned in this book, is not a solitary pursuit of immortality; rather, it's a holistic path to enriching our lives, extending our vitality, and nurturing our connection to the universal life force. This is a path where spiritual growth and physical well-being intertwine, leading to a more fulfilling and longer journey in this earthly realm. The evidence linking meditation and telomere length adds another layer to this journey, offering a scientific perspective on the profound benefits of a practice long embraced for its spiritual significance. The future undoubtedly holds even more discoveries regarding the connection between meditation and longevity. As research continues to unveil the intricate mechanisms involved, we will gain a deeper appreciation for this powerful tool in our quest for a healthier, more fulfilling, and longer life.

The Impact of Meditation on Hormonal Balance

The remarkable influence of meditation extends beyond the cellular level, impacting the intricate symphony of our endocrine system and its hormonal orchestra. Our hormones, the chemical messengers that orchestrate countless bodily functions, play a pivotal role in our overall health and longevity. Chronic stress, a pervasive feature of modern life, often disrupts this delicate hormonal balance, leading to a cascade of negative consequences. Meditation, however, offers a potent antidote, a means of restoring harmony and equilibrium to this vital system.

One of the most significant ways meditation impacts hormonal balance is through its profound effect on the hypothalamic-pituitary-adrenal (HPA) axis. This axis, a crucial component of our stress response system, governs the release of cortisol, the primary stress hormone. Under chronic stress, the HPA axis can become dysregulated, leading to elevated cortisol levels. This sustained elevation contributes to a range of adverse effects, including weight gain, impaired immunity, increased inflammation, and even an increased risk of cardiovascular disease.

Meditation, particularly mindfulness meditation, has been shown to modulate the activity of the HPA axis, reducing the secretion of cortisol and mitigating the negative consequences of chronic stress. Studies employing various neuroimaging techniques have revealed that regular meditation practice can lead to structural and functional changes in the brain regions associated with stress response, including the amygdala and prefrontal cortex. The amygdala, often referred to as the brain's fear center, is responsible for triggering the stress response. Meditation helps to downregulate its activity, reducing the intensity of the stress response. Meanwhile, the prefrontal cortex, involved in executive functions such as self-regulation and emotional control, strengthens its influence over the amygdala, enabling a more measured and balanced response to stressors.

The positive impact of meditation on cortisol levels isn't merely a matter of reducing its overproduction; it's also about facilitating a more balanced and adaptable hormonal response. Instead of a constant state of high alert, the body learns to respond more appropriately to challenges, avoiding the chronic elevation of cortisol that undermines health. This improved adaptability translates to greater resilience in the face of stress, an essential element of maintaining both physical and mental well-being. Individuals who regularly practice meditation are better equipped to navigate life's inevitable stressors without experiencing the detrimental effects of prolonged cortisol exposure.

Beyond cortisol, meditation's influence extends to other crucial hormones. For example, it has been associated with increased levels of dehydroepiandrosterone (DHEA), often referred to as the "anti-aging hormone." DHEA plays a significant role in various bodily functions, including immune response, energy production, and cognitive function. Maintaining healthy levels of DHEA is essential for preserving vitality and combating age-related decline. Meditation's ability to boost DHEA levels adds another layer to its anti-aging effects.

Furthermore, meditation has been linked to improved levels of other hormones, such as testosterone and estrogen. These sex hormones, crucial for reproductive health and overall well-being, can become imbalanced under chronic stress. By reducing stress and promoting a state of equilibrium, meditation contributes to maintaining a healthy hormonal balance. Studies have suggested that regular meditation can improve sexual function and libido, potentially linked to the regulation of these hormones. However, it's important to note that this is an area that requires further research to establish concrete conclusions.

The benefits of a balanced hormonal profile extend far beyond specific hormones. They contribute to a holistic sense of well-being, impacting various aspects of our physical and mental health. A balanced hormonal system enhances immune function, promotes healthy sleep patterns, improves mood and cognitive function, and supports overall vitality. By cultivating a harmonious hormonal environment through meditation, we lay the groundwork for a healthier, more vibrant, and longer life.

Beyond the direct effects on hormone levels, meditation also influences our hormonal balance indirectly through its impact on other physiological systems. For instance, meditation has been shown to reduce inflammation throughout the body. Chronic inflammation is implicated in a multitude of age-related diseases, and meditation's ability to counteract it is a significant factor in its contribution to longevity. By reducing inflammation, meditation indirectly helps to maintain healthy hormone levels and prevent hormonal imbalances that could lead to health problems.

Meditation's impact on the autonomic nervous system also contributes to its beneficial effects on hormonal balance. The autonomic nervous system controls involuntary bodily functions, such as heart rate, breathing, and digestion. Chronic stress can lead to an overactivation of the sympathetic nervous system, the "fight-or-flight" response, causing an imbalance in the autonomic nervous system. This imbalance can result in elevated stress hormones and other negative physiological consequences.

Meditation, however, promotes the activation of the parasympathetic nervous system, the "rest-and-digest" response, counteracting the effects of chronic stress. This activation leads to a calming effect on the body, reducing heart rate and blood pressure, and promoting relaxation and digestive health. This shift towards parasympathetic dominance is crucial for maintaining hormonal balance and overall well-being.

The improved sleep quality often associated with meditation also contributes to hormonal regulation. During sleep, our bodies produce and regulate various hormones, and disrupted sleep can lead to hormonal imbalances. Meditation's ability to improve sleep quality, by calming the mind and reducing stress, promotes healthy hormone production and regulation. This, in turn, contributes to overall health and well-being, playing a significant role in extending lifespan.

The science of meditation's impact on hormonal balance is still an evolving field of research. However, the accumulated evidence clearly demonstrates a significant connection. Through its influence on the HPA axis, its ability to modulate stress hormones, and its indirect effects on inflammation, sleep, and the autonomic nervous system, meditation offers a powerful tool for maintaining hormonal balance and promoting overall health and longevity. As research continues, we can expect to further uncover the intricate mechanisms involved and gain a deeper understanding of this remarkable mind-body connection. The integration of meditation into our lives, therefore, is not merely a spiritual practice but a proactive measure for safeguarding our health and enhancing our potential to live longer, healthier, and more fulfilling lives. The holistic path to longevity, as presented in this book, embraces the multifaceted benefits of meditation, highlighting its crucial role in achieving a balanced hormonal system and thus extending our vitality and our connection with the life force that sustains us. The journey towards spiritual enlightenment, therefore, becomes interwoven with the very fabric of our physical well-being, making our pursuit of immortality of the soul a truly holistic endeavor.

Boosting the Immune System Through Meditation

The profound impact of meditation extends beyond the endocrine system, reaching into the very core of our body's defense mechanisms: the immune system. Our immune system, a complex network of cells and organs, acts as our vigilant guardian, constantly patrolling our bodies, identifying and neutralizing harmful invaders like viruses, bacteria, and other pathogens. Maintaining a robust immune system is paramount to our overall health and longevity, and meditation, surprisingly, plays a significant role in bolstering these defenses.

Modern life, with its relentless pace and constant barrage of stressors, often compromises the efficiency of our immune system. Chronic stress, a prevalent ailment of our time, triggers a cascade of physiological responses that weaken our ability to fight off disease. The body's stress response, orchestrated by the hypothalamic-pituitary-adrenal (HPA) axis, releases hormones like cortisol, which, while beneficial in short bursts, can become detrimental when chronically elevated. Prolonged exposure to high cortisol levels suppresses the immune system, leaving us vulnerable to infections and illnesses.

Meditation, however, offers a powerful countermeasure to this chronic stress response. Through consistent practice, meditation cultivates a state of deep relaxation and inner calm, effectively mitigating the negative impacts of stress on the immune system. Studies have demonstrated that regular meditation can significantly lower cortisol levels, restoring hormonal balance and allowing the immune system to function optimally.

The mechanisms by which meditation enhances immune function are multifaceted and complex. One key pathway involves the modulation of the autonomic nervous system (ANS), the system responsible for regulating involuntary bodily functions such as heart rate, breathing, and digestion. The ANS is comprised of two branches: the sympathetic nervous system (SNS), associated with the "fight-or-flight" response, and the parasympathetic nervous system (PNS), responsible for the "rest-and-digest" response. Chronic stress activates the SNS, leading to increased heart rate, blood pressure, and cortisol release. Conversely, meditation activates the PNS, promoting relaxation, lowering heart rate and blood pressure, and reducing cortisol levels. This shift towards PNS dominance creates an environment conducive to immune system restoration.

Furthermore, meditation's influence extends to the cellular level, impacting the activity and function of immune cells such as lymphocytes, macrophages, and natural killer (NK) cells. These cells are the frontline defenders of our immune system, playing crucial roles in identifying and eliminating pathogens. Research suggests that meditation can increase the activity and number of these immune cells, thereby enhancing the body's ability to fight off infections. Studies have shown that individuals who regularly practice meditation exhibit increased NK cell activity, indicating a heightened capacity to destroy cancer cells and viruses.

The impact of meditation on inflammation is another critical aspect of its immune-boosting effects. Inflammation, while a necessary part of the body's healing process, can become chronic and damaging when prolonged. Chronic inflammation is implicated in numerous diseases, including heart disease, autoimmune disorders, and cancer. Meditation, through its stress-reducing effects and its ability to modulate the HPA axis, has been shown to reduce inflammation markers in the body. By dampening the inflammatory response, meditation helps protect the body from the damaging effects of chronic inflammation, thus contributing to overall health and longevity.

Beyond its physiological effects, meditation fosters a holistic approach to well-being, addressing the mind-body connection crucial for immune function. Stress, as we've discussed, negatively impacts the immune system. But stress isn't just a physiological response; it's also a mental and emotional state. Meditation provides tools to manage stress not just on a physical level, but also on a mental and emotional level. By cultivating inner peace, mindfulness, and emotional regulation, meditation empowers individuals to better cope with life's challenges, reducing the overall stress load on the body and, in turn, bolstering the immune system.

The evidence supporting the link between meditation and immune function is growing steadily, with numerous studies demonstrating positive effects across various populations and meditation techniques. These studies employ a range of methodologies, including measuring immune cell activity, analyzing inflammatory markers, and assessing self-reported health outcomes. While the exact mechanisms are still being explored, the consistent findings indicate a clear and significant relationship between meditation and enhanced immunity.

Consider, for example, research conducted on mindfulness-based stress reduction (MBSR) programs. These programs, which typically involve a combination of meditation, yoga, and mindful movement, have consistently shown to improve immune function in participants. Studies have documented significant increases in NK cell activity, reduced levels of inflammatory markers, and improved self-reported health in individuals who participated in MBSR programs. Similar results have been observed in studies focusing on other meditation techniques, such as transcendental meditation (TM) and loving-kindness meditation.

The benefits of meditation extend beyond the immediate impact on the immune system. By cultivating a state of inner peace and reducing stress, meditation fosters a holistic sense of well-being that promotes healthy lifestyle choices. Individuals who meditate are often more likely to engage in regular exercise, maintain a healthy diet, and prioritize sufficient sleep, all of which further contribute to a strong immune system. This synergistic effect of meditation, coupled with healthy lifestyle choices, creates a powerful combination for maximizing overall health and longevity.

The integration of meditation into one's life is not just a spiritual practice; it is a proactive investment in one's physical and mental health. The evidence convincingly demonstrates that regular meditation enhances immune function, reducing vulnerability to disease and promoting overall well-being. By incorporating meditation into daily routines, individuals empower themselves to build resilience against stress, nurture a robust immune system, and embark on a path towards a healthier, longer, and more fulfilling life, thereby enhancing the pursuit of the immortality of the soul. This holistic approach aligns perfectly with the broader philosophy of this book, emphasizing the interconnectedness of mind, body, and spirit in the journey towards spiritual and physical longevity. The path to a vibrant, disease-resistant body is not solely defined by diet and exercise; it is enriched by the inner peace and harmony cultivated through the consistent practice of meditation, a practice that nurtures both the physical and spiritual aspects of our being.

The science is increasingly revealing the intricate interplay between mental and physical health, underscoring the importance of holistic well-being. Meditation serves as a powerful bridge, connecting these seemingly disparate aspects of our existence. It is not simply a tool for stress reduction; it is a gateway to unlocking the body's innate ability to heal and thrive, a cornerstone of a longer, healthier, and more meaningful life. The implications extend beyond the individual, impacting families and communities. By promoting mental and physical resilience, meditation has the potential to create healthier, more harmonious societies. It's an investment in the future, both individually and collectively, fostering a world where well-being is not just a goal, but a vibrant reality. This comprehensive approach to health and well-being, rooted in the principles of mind-body connection and the transformative power of meditation, forms a vital pillar in our pursuit of a longer, healthier, and more spiritually fulfilling existence, bringing us closer to the concept of the immortality of the soul. As we further explore the depths of this connection, we unlock not just improved physical health but also a deeper understanding of our own inner potential, guiding us towards a more harmonious and fulfilling life. The practice of meditation, therefore, transcends the realm of simple wellness strategies; it represents a profound journey of self-discovery and empowerment, interwoven with the very fabric of our pursuit of spiritual and physical longevity. The subtle shifts in our inner landscape, mirrored by measurable changes in our physiology, demonstrate the profound power of integrating mind and body, culminating in a healthier, more resilient, and ultimately more spiritually aligned existence.

Meditation and Cardiovascular Health

The remarkable interconnectedness of mind and body, so profoundly illuminated by the impact of meditation on the immune system, extends equally to the cardiovascular system. Our hearts, the tireless engines of our lives, are not merely physical pumps; they are deeply susceptible to the rhythms of our minds. Chronic stress, anxiety, and negative emotions significantly contribute to cardiovascular disease, the leading cause of death globally. Meditation, by its very nature, offers a powerful antidote to this pervasive modern affliction.

Numerous scientific studies have demonstrated the beneficial effects of meditation on various cardiovascular parameters. Research consistently shows a reduction in blood pressure among individuals who regularly practice meditation. This is not merely a superficial effect; rather, it reflects a deeper, more systemic modulation of the body's physiological response to stress. When confronted with stressful situations, our bodies typically release hormones like adrenaline and cortisol, leading to an increase in heart rate and blood pressure. Meditation, through its calming influence on the nervous system, helps to mitigate this hyper-reactive response. It allows the body to return to a state of homeostasis more efficiently, reducing the strain on the cardiovascular system.

One of the key mechanisms through which meditation achieves this is the activation of the parasympathetic nervous system, often referred to as the "rest and digest" system. This counterbalances the sympathetic nervous system, responsible for the "fight or flight" response. By cultivating a state of calm and relaxation, meditation strengthens the parasympathetic nervous system's influence, promoting a slower heart rate, lower blood pressure, and reduced vascular resistance. This, in turn, translates to a decreased risk of hypertension, atherosclerosis, and other cardiovascular complications.

The impact of meditation extends beyond blood pressure regulation. Studies have also shown its beneficial effects on heart rate variability (HRV). HRV refers to the variation in the time intervals between heartbeats. A higher HRV is generally associated with better cardiovascular health and resilience to stress. Meditation has been shown to increase HRV, indicating a greater adaptability and responsiveness of the cardiovascular system. This improved adaptability enables the heart to respond more effectively to changing demands, further reducing the risk of cardiovascular events.

Furthermore, meditation has been linked to a reduction in inflammatory markers associated with cardiovascular disease. Inflammation plays a crucial role in the development and progression of atherosclerosis, a condition characterized by the buildup of plaque in the arteries. Chronic inflammation, often driven by stress and unhealthy lifestyle choices, can contribute to the formation of these plaques, leading to heart attacks and strokes. Meditation, by its stress-reducing and calming effects, helps to dampen this inflammatory response, potentially mitigating the risk of atherosclerosis.

The positive effects of meditation on cardiovascular health are not limited to specific techniques. Different forms of meditation, such as mindfulness meditation, transcendental meditation, and yoga-based meditation, have all demonstrated similar cardiovascular benefits. This suggests that the core mechanism underlying these benefits is the cultivation of a state of mental calm and relaxation, rather than the specific techniques employed. The consistency and regularity of the practice appear to be more significant factors than the specific type of meditation.

The scientific evidence supporting these claims is substantial. Meta-analyses, which combine the results of multiple studies, have consistently demonstrated the positive effects of meditation on blood pressure, HRV, and inflammatory markers. These analyses have helped to solidify the understanding of the mechanisms by which meditation improves cardiovascular health and to establish meditation as a valuable complementary therapy in the management of cardiovascular risk factors.

Beyond the quantitative data, the qualitative experiences of individuals who practice meditation offer further compelling evidence. Many report a significant reduction in stress and anxiety levels, accompanied by an increased sense of calm and well-being. These subjective experiences, while not directly quantifiable, reflect a profound shift in the individual's relationship with their body and their response to stress. This shift, in itself, contributes to a healthier cardiovascular profile.

However, it is crucial to emphasize that meditation should not be considered a replacement for conventional medical treatment of cardiovascular disease. Individuals with existing cardiovascular conditions should continue to follow their physician's recommendations and adhere to prescribed medications. Meditation should be viewed as a complementary therapy that can enhance the effectiveness of conventional treatments and improve overall well-being.

The integration of meditation into a holistic approach to cardiovascular health offers a promising avenue for improving both physical and mental well-being. By combining meditation with other healthy lifestyle choices, such as regular exercise, a balanced diet, and adequate sleep, individuals can significantly reduce their risk of cardiovascular disease and enhance their overall quality of life. This integrated approach acknowledges the inseparable connection between mind and body, recognizing that the health of one is intrinsically linked to the health of the other.

Moreover, the accessibility and cost-effectiveness of meditation make it a valuable tool for promoting cardiovascular health across populations. Unlike many other therapeutic interventions, meditation requires no specialized equipment or expensive medications. It can be practiced virtually anywhere, at any time, making it a readily accessible tool for improving cardiovascular health regardless of socioeconomic status.

The growing body of scientific evidence, coupled with the widespread anecdotal reports of improved well-being, underscores the importance of incorporating meditation into a comprehensive strategy for promoting cardiovascular health and longevity. It is not merely a stress-reduction technique; it is a profound pathway towards a healthier, more balanced, and more spiritually fulfilling life, bringing us closer to the enduring essence of the soul. The synergistic effects of meditation, when combined with other healthy lifestyle choices, offer a powerful and holistic approach to preventative healthcare, offering individuals the opportunity to take proactive steps towards a longer and healthier life, a journey towards the immortality of the soul. The subtle shifts in heart rate, blood pressure, and overall cardiovascular functioning reflect the profound, transformative power of connecting mind and body, a journey that transcends the physical and touches upon the very essence of our being. This holistic approach to health and longevity, integrating the science of meditation with the wisdom of spiritual practice, offers a powerful pathway towards a richer, more fulfilling life, extending far beyond the limitations of the physical realm.

Developing Empathy and Understanding Through Meditation

The capacity for empathy, for truly understanding and feeling the emotions of others, is a cornerstone of a compassionate and fulfilling life. It's a quality often undervalued in our fast-paced, often individualistic world, yet it forms the very bedrock of meaningful connection and lasting peace. While we may intellectually grasp the concept of empathy, cultivating it within ourselves requires dedicated practice and a willingness to delve into the depths of our own emotional landscape. Meditation provides a powerful tool for this transformative journey.

Meditation isn't simply about silencing the mind; it's about cultivating a profound awareness of both our inner world and the world around us. This awareness extends to others, allowing us to see beyond the surface, to perceive the subtle nuances of their experiences, their joys and sorrows, their hopes and fears. Through consistent meditation, we begin to recognize the interconnectedness of all beings. We realize that we are not isolated entities, but rather threads in the rich tapestry of life, inextricably linked to one another through shared experiences and a common humanity.

This sense of interconnectedness is not a mere philosophical concept; it's a visceral feeling, a deep knowing that resonates within our being. When we meditate, we quiet the incessant chatter of the mind, the constant stream of thoughts and judgments that often prevent us from truly seeing others. As the mind stills, a space opens, a space of receptivity and openness to the experiences of those around us. We begin to perceive the world, not through our own limited perspectives, but through a lens of compassion and understanding.

Consider, for instance, the experience of observing someone struggling with a difficult situation. Without meditation, our initial reaction might be one of judgment, perhaps even indifference. We may rush to conclusions, make assumptions about their circumstances, or simply dismiss their plight as irrelevant to our own lives. However, when we approach such a situation with a meditative mindset, we cultivate a different response. Instead of judging, we observe. Instead of assuming, we seek to understand.

In a meditative state, our awareness expands beyond our own immediate concerns. We become more attuned to the subtle cues and expressions of those around us. We notice the tremor in their voice, the tightness in their shoulders, the sadness in their eyes. These subtle signals, often missed in the whirlwind of daily life, become profoundly meaningful. They reveal the underlying emotions, the hidden struggles, the vulnerability that lies beneath the surface.

This enhanced awareness fosters empathy. We begin to see ourselves reflected in the experiences of others, recognizing the shared human condition that binds us together. We remember our own moments of struggle, our own times of vulnerability, our own experiences of pain and loss. This shared human experience forms a powerful bridge of connection, allowing us to approach others with compassion, understanding, and support.

The practice of loving-kindness meditation, in particular, is incredibly effective in cultivating empathy. This involves sending out feelings of warmth, kindness, and compassion to ourselves and then extending those feelings to others, starting with loved ones and gradually expanding to include strangers, even those we may find difficult to connect with. The consistent repetition of these loving-kindness phrases – "May you be well, may you be happy, may you be peaceful, may you be free from suffering" – helps to open our hearts and cultivate a deep sense of interconnectedness.

This is not a passive process. Cultivating empathy through meditation requires active engagement. It demands that we confront our own prejudices, our own biases, our own preconceived notions about others. It requires that we challenge our own emotional responses and strive to see things from another's perspective. This is not always easy. It may require confronting uncomfortable truths about ourselves and the world around us.

For example, imagine encountering someone who holds radically different views from your own. Your immediate response may be anger, frustration, or even disgust. Meditation provides a path toward a more constructive response. By slowing down, quieting the mind, and connecting with your own center, you can create space for compassion and understanding. Instead of resorting to defensiveness or argument, you can try to understand the other person's perspective, to empathize with their feelings, even if you don't agree with their beliefs.

This process of active empathy can be profoundly transformative. It leads not only to improved relationships and more fulfilling connections, but also to a deeper understanding of yourself. By cultivating compassion for others, we are in effect cultivating compassion for ourselves. We learn to be more forgiving, more understanding, and more accepting, both of our own imperfections and the imperfections of those around us.

Through regular meditation practice, we can train our minds to move beyond the limitations of our own ego-centric perspectives. We become less self-absorbed and more attuned to the needs and experiences of others. This leads to more compassionate actions, more meaningful interactions, and a deeper sense of belonging. The world becomes a richer, more vibrant place, filled with genuine connection and shared humanity.

Moreover, the cultivation of empathy extends beyond our interpersonal relationships. It informs our interactions with the wider world, influencing our political views, our economic choices, and our commitment to social justice. When we understand the suffering of others, we are more likely to act in ways that alleviate that suffering. We become advocates for change, agents of compassion, and builders of a more just and equitable world.

The journey toward cultivating empathy through meditation is a lifelong process. It's not a destination, but a path of continuous growth and learning. It demands patience, persistence, and a willingness to embrace the challenges along the way. But the rewards are immeasurable – a deeper understanding of ourselves and others, a more compassionate heart, and a life filled with genuine connection and lasting peace. The ability to see ourselves reflected in the lives of others, to feel their joys and sorrows as if they were our own, is the ultimate expression of human connection, a testament to the power of empathy, and a gift we can cultivate through the practice of meditation. It is, in essence, a step towards a more loving and harmonious world, and a path toward the spiritual growth that leads to a more fulfilling and meaningful existence. The very act of extending compassion, understanding, and empathy to those around us helps us to nurture those same qualities within ourselves, creating a virtuous cycle of growth and transformation. This internal shift, fostered through dedicated meditation practice, is what ultimately empowers us to live a life imbued with compassion and understanding, a life that truly reflects the interconnectedness of all beings. This inner transformation is not merely a personal benefit; it is a contribution to the greater good, a ripple effect of positivity that touches the lives of those around us and helps to build a more peaceful and harmonious world.

Overcoming Anger and Cultivating Forgiveness

Anger, a potent emotion often perceived as destructive, can, when understood and managed correctly, become a catalyst for profound self-discovery and spiritual growth. It is a signal, a visceral alarm bell alerting us to unmet needs, perceived injustices, or a violation of our boundaries. To simply suppress anger is to ignore a crucial message from our inner selves. Instead, we must learn to listen to this message, understand its origins, and transform its destructive energy into something constructive. This process begins with acknowledging the validity of our anger, without judgment or self-criticism. It's okay to feel angry; it's a natural human emotion. The key is in how we choose to respond to that anger.

Meditation offers a powerful tool for navigating the tempestuous waters of anger. Through focused breathwork and mindful observation, we can learn to detach from the immediate grip of anger, creating space between the triggering event and our reactive response. Imagine anger as a wave crashing against the shore. Initially, the wave's power is overwhelming, but with time, we learn that the wave eventually recedes, leaving the shore intact. Meditation allows us to observe this wave, to witness its rise and fall without being swept away by its force. By focusing on our breath, we anchor ourselves in the present moment, preventing our minds from being hijacked by the narratives and justifications that often accompany anger. This mindful observation allows for a gradual reduction in the intensity of the emotion, creating space for a more balanced and rational response.

A crucial aspect of overcoming anger involves understanding its root causes. Often, anger masks deeper emotions, such as fear, sadness, or vulnerability. These underlying emotions may stem from past traumas, unmet needs, or ingrained beliefs. Through introspection and meditation, we can uncover these root causes, allowing us to address them directly. Journaling can be a valuable tool in this process, providing a space to explore our feelings without judgment. By writing down our thoughts and emotions related to a specific instance of anger, we can begin to identify patterns and triggers, leading to a greater understanding of ourselves and our emotional responses. This self-awareness is crucial in preventing future episodes of anger. Meditation, with its focus on self-reflection, facilitates this process of introspection, allowing us to gain a deeper understanding of our own emotional landscape.

Forgiveness, often misunderstood as condoning harmful actions, is actually a profound act of self-liberation. Holding onto resentment and anger consumes our energy, clouding our judgment and preventing us from moving forward. Forgiveness, in this context, is not about excusing the actions of others, but rather about releasing ourselves from the emotional burden of carrying the weight of past hurts. It's about choosing to break free from the cycle of negativity and reclaim our inner peace. This process begins with acknowledging the pain caused by the hurtful actions, allowing ourselves to feel the emotions without judgment. Then, through mindful meditation, we gradually shift our focus from the pain to a place of compassion, both for ourselves and for the person who caused the hurt. Recognizing the human fallibility inherent in all of us, including those who have wronged us, can aid this process. Understanding that their actions might have stemmed from their own pain, fear, or ignorance can foster a sense of empathy, which is essential for true forgiveness.

The practice of loving-kindness meditation can be particularly helpful in cultivating forgiveness. This technique involves directing feelings of love and compassion towards ourselves, then extending these feelings to others, including those who have harmed us. By silently repeating phrases such as "May you be happy, may you be healthy, may you be peaceful," we cultivate a sense of warmth and goodwill towards them, gradually releasing the grip of resentment. This isn't about instantly erasing the hurt, but about choosing to move beyond it, towards a state of inner peace and freedom. This compassionate approach helps to transform the anger into empathy, fostering healing and releasing the emotional burden we carry.

Forgiveness does not necessitate reconciliation or interaction with the person who caused the hurt. Forgiveness is a personal journey, an internal shift that releases us from the grip of negativity. It is a gift we give ourselves, allowing us to heal and move forward. The process is not linear; it's iterative, involving setbacks and progress. It is a practice, requiring patience and compassion with ourselves along the way.

Specific techniques can facilitate the process of overcoming anger and cultivating forgiveness. One effective technique involves visualizing the person who caused the hurt and sending them feelings of compassion and understanding. Imagine their pain, their struggles, and their reasons for acting as they did. This process isn't about diminishing the harm done, but about expanding our perspective, gaining a deeper understanding of their motivations, and thus releasing the grip of anger. It allows for a shift in focus from condemnation to compassion.

Another useful practice is the "compassion break". Throughout the day, when anger arises, take a moment to pause, breathe deeply, and shift your focus from the anger to your own well-being. Acknowledge the emotion, but choose not to be overwhelmed by it. Engage in self-compassion, acknowledging the validity of your feelings, but choosing to respond in a way that nourishes your well-being instead of exacerbating your anger. This practice takes discipline and consistent effort, but it yields significant results in managing anger effectively.

Beyond these individual practices, consider the larger context of your life. Are you engaging in activities that support your well-being? Are you getting enough rest, engaging in physical activity, and nurturing supportive relationships? Chronic stress, exhaustion, and social isolation can significantly heighten our reactivity and increase our susceptibility to anger. Addressing these underlying factors through lifestyle changes, such as prioritizing self-care, regular exercise, and mindfulness practices, helps create a more resilient foundation for managing emotions.

Furthermore, cultivating self-compassion is vital. We are all imperfect beings, prone to making mistakes and experiencing negative emotions. Rather than berating ourselves for feeling angry, we should approach these emotions with understanding and self-acceptance. Self-criticism only exacerbates negative emotions, creating a vicious cycle of negativity. By treating ourselves with the same compassion we extend to others, we create a supportive environment for emotional growth and healing.

In conclusion, overcoming anger and cultivating forgiveness are not one-time events but ongoing practices, requiring patience, persistence, and self-compassion. Through meditation, introspection, and the conscious cultivation of empathy and loving-kindness, we can transform anger from a destructive force into a catalyst for growth and spiritual awakening. By releasing the grip of resentment, we create space for peace, joy, and a deeper connection with ourselves and the world around us. This journey of self-discovery leads to a more fulfilling life, enriched by compassion and understanding, ultimately aligning with the path toward the immortality of the soul. The ability to forgive, to release the burden of anger, is a powerful act of self-love, a testament to our capacity for growth, and a crucial step towards living a life imbued with peace and spiritual fulfillment. This process of transformation, deeply connected to our spiritual journey, allows us to move beyond the limitations of the ego and embrace the boundless potential of our true selves.

Building Healthy Relationships Through Mindfulness

Building healthy relationships hinges on our ability to connect authentically with others, and this connection is profoundly enhanced by cultivating mindfulness. Mindfulness, the practice of paying attention to the present moment without judgment, acts as a bridge, connecting us not only to ourselves but also to those we share our lives with. It allows us to perceive our relationships with greater clarity, empathy, and compassion, fostering a deeper understanding and appreciation for the intricate dance of human connection.

The cornerstone of mindful relating lies in conscious communication. Often, we communicate reactively, driven by ingrained patterns, unexamined assumptions, and emotional baggage. This reactive communication can lead to misunderstandings, conflict, and emotional distance. Mindfulness, however, empowers us to pause, to breathe, and to choose our responses consciously. Instead of reacting impulsively, we can observe our emotions, our thoughts, and the other person's perspective before we speak. This pause allows us to respond with greater clarity, empathy, and respect.

Consider a typical scenario: a disagreement arises between partners. In a non-mindful interaction, accusations fly, voices rise, and resentment builds. Each partner is trapped in their own emotional narrative, unable to see the other's perspective. However, if both partners approach the disagreement with mindfulness, the dynamic shifts dramatically. They begin by acknowledging their own emotions, perhaps noticing the tightness in their chest or the rising tension in their shoulders. They listen attentively to their partner, seeking to understand their perspective, even if they don't agree with it. They practice empathy, trying to step into their partner's shoes and understand their feelings. This shift from reaction to response transforms the interaction from a battleground into a space for dialogue and understanding.

Mindfulness also helps us to cultivate patience and tolerance in our relationships. Relationships are not static; they are dynamic systems constantly evolving and adapting. There will be moments of friction, misunderstandings, and challenges. Mindfulness allows us to navigate these moments with grace and patience, recognizing that conflict is not necessarily a sign of failure but rather an opportunity for growth and deeper connection. Instead of becoming reactive and defensive, we can view challenges as opportunities to deepen our self-awareness and strengthen our ability to communicate effectively.

Furthermore, mindfulness encourages us to appreciate the small, everyday moments of connection. Often, we are so caught up in our thoughts and to-do lists that we fail to notice the simple joys of being with loved ones. Mindfulness helps us to be fully present, to savour the warmth of a hug, the sound of a loved one's laughter, or the shared silence of a peaceful evening. These moments, when fully appreciated, strengthen the bonds of love and connection. By practicing mindful appreciation, we cultivate gratitude for the presence of others in our lives, reinforcing the positive aspects of our relationships.

The practice of loving-kindness meditation can profoundly enhance our capacity for empathy and compassion in our relationships. Loving-kindness meditation involves extending feelings of warmth, compassion, and kindness towards ourselves and others. We begin by directing these feelings towards ourselves, recognizing our inherent worth and compassionately acknowledging our imperfections. Then, we extend these feelings to loved ones, friends, neutral individuals, and eventually even those we find challenging. This practice cultivates a sense of interconnectedness, reminding us that we are all part of a larger web of life, sharing similar hopes, fears, and aspirations.

This practice isn't simply about feeling positive emotions; it's about cultivating a deep sense of understanding and empathy for others. When we practice loving-kindness meditation, we begin to see ourselves and others with greater clarity, recognizing the shared humanity that binds us together. This deeper understanding fosters greater compassion, allowing us to approach our relationships with kindness, patience, and understanding, even in moments of conflict or disagreement. It allows us to see beyond the surface, to recognize the underlying needs and vulnerabilities of those around us.

Active listening, a cornerstone of mindful communication, goes beyond simply hearing words. It involves fully engaging with the speaker, paying attention not only to their words but also to their body language, tone of voice, and emotional state. It requires setting aside our own thoughts and agendas, creating a safe space for the other person to express themselves without judgment or interruption. This requires concentration and a willingness to truly understand the other person's perspective, even if it differs from our own.

When we listen mindfully, we are not just hearing words; we are witnessing the human experience. We are connecting with another person at a deeper level, recognizing their vulnerabilities and empathizing with their struggles. Active listening strengthens relationships by creating a sense of being truly heard and understood. It fosters a sense of trust and intimacy, allowing for open communication and a deeper connection between individuals. It is an act of profound respect and acknowledgment of the other's inherent worth.

Mindfulness also plays a crucial role in managing conflict constructively. Disagreements are inevitable in any relationship, but how we handle them determines the health and longevity of the connection. A mindful approach to conflict involves acknowledging the emotions involved, both our own and our partner's, without judgment or defensiveness. It involves clearly expressing our needs and feelings, using "I" statements to avoid blame and accusation. It means listening actively to our partner's perspective, seeking to understand their point of view, even if we disagree with it.

Mindful conflict resolution is not about winning or losing; it's about finding common ground and solutions that work for both parties. It involves a willingness to compromise and to find creative solutions that address everyone's needs. This approach requires patience, empathy, and a commitment to understanding the other person's perspective. The ultimate goal is not to eliminate conflict altogether but to navigate it constructively, strengthening the bond between individuals rather than damaging it.

Furthermore, the practice of self-compassion is integral to building healthy relationships. Before we can offer compassion to others, we must first cultivate compassion for ourselves. Self-compassion involves treating ourselves with the same kindness, understanding, and forgiveness we would offer a close friend. It means acknowledging our imperfections without self-criticism, recognizing that everyone makes mistakes, and that these mistakes are not a reflection of our inherent worth.

When we practice self-compassion, we become more resilient and less prone to defensiveness in our relationships. We are better able to handle criticism and conflict without taking things personally, recognizing that our partners' reactions often stem from their own experiences and emotional baggage. Self-compassion allows us to approach our relationships with greater humility and understanding, fostering a sense of mutual respect and empathy.

In essence, mindfulness is not a quick fix for relationship problems but rather a transformative practice that cultivates the inner qualities necessary for building healthy, fulfilling relationships. It empowers us to communicate more effectively, to manage conflict constructively, to cultivate empathy and compassion, and to appreciate the simple joys of human connection. By incorporating mindfulness into our daily lives, we create space for authentic connection, strengthening the bonds of love and understanding, and ultimately enriching our lives in profound ways. This journey of self-discovery through mindfulness aligns perfectly with the pursuit of spiritual growth and the immortality of the soul, as a life enriched by loving connections contributes to a richer and more meaningful existence, extending beyond the physical realm. The peace and understanding fostered within ourselves through meditation and mindfulness naturally radiate outward, enriching our interactions and deepening our bonds with others, creating a ripple effect of positivity that strengthens our spiritual journey.

Extending Compassion to All Beings

The cultivation of love and compassion, as we've explored, begins within, a blossoming that gradually extends its tendrils outward, enriching our connections with others. However, the true scope of compassion transcends the boundaries of human interaction. It encompasses a boundless, all-encompassing love that extends to every sentient being, a recognition of the interconnected web of life that binds us all. This universal compassion, this expansive empathy, is not merely a desirable virtue; it's a fundamental aspect of spiritual evolution, a crucial step towards the immortality of the soul.

When we limit our compassion to our immediate circle – family, friends, colleagues – we confine its potential. We fail to recognize the inherent worth and dignity of all living creatures, the shared breath of life that animates each and every one. To truly cultivate compassion, we must expand our circle of empathy, embracing animals, plants, and even the seemingly inanimate elements of nature. This is not a matter of sentimentality or anthropomorphism, but a deeper understanding of the interconnectedness of existence.

Consider the intricate dance of life unfolding around us. The sun nourishes the plants, the plants sustain the animals, and the animals, in turn, contribute to the delicate balance of ecosystems. Each element plays a crucial role, each contributing to the harmonious symphony of life. To disregard any part of this symphony, to diminish the importance of any living being, is to disrupt the balance, to diminish the richness of the whole. To cultivate universal compassion is to appreciate this interconnectedness, to recognize the intrinsic value of every living creature, from the smallest insect to the largest whale.

This expansion of compassion requires a shift in perspective, a movement away from anthropocentric viewpoints. We must move beyond the limited lens that places humans at the center of the universe, recognizing instead our place within a larger, more expansive reality. This shift involves acknowledging the suffering of other beings – the pain of a wounded animal, the slow death of a plant deprived of sunlight, the vulnerability of a creature threatened by extinction. It is in acknowledging this suffering, in feeling it resonate within our own hearts, that true compassion blossoms.

The practice of meditation provides a powerful tool for cultivating this universal compassion. Through focused attention and deep relaxation, we can quiet the mind's incessant chatter and connect with the deeper, more intuitive aspects of our being. In this state of stillness, we can access a wellspring of empathy, allowing the suffering of others to touch us, to move us to action. We can visualize the interconnectedness of all life, picturing the web that connects us all, and feel the compassion flow outward from our hearts, extending to every creature, large and small.

This is not a passive act of feeling; it's an active practice. It involves making conscious choices to align our actions with our values. It might mean choosing to be a vegetarian or vegan, minimizing our impact on the environment, supporting organizations dedicated to animal welfare or environmental protection, or simply showing kindness and respect to every living being we encounter. These actions are not merely symbolic gestures; they are tangible expressions of our deepened compassion, concrete manifestations of our expanding circle of empathy.

Think of the countless ways in which we can extend this compassion. A simple act of kindness towards a stray animal – offering food and water, seeking veterinary care if needed – can have a profound impact. Similarly, tending to a garden, nurturing plants with care and attention, is an act of compassion, a recognition of the life force that animates even the seemingly inanimate. Even the seemingly small actions – refraining from littering, conserving water, choosing sustainable products – contribute to a larger picture of collective responsibility, a testament to our growing capacity for universal love.

The spiritual path, the journey towards the immortality of the soul, is not a solitary pursuit. It's a path of interconnectedness, a journey that involves extending our love and compassion to all beings. Our actions ripple outward, impacting not only ourselves but the world around us. By cultivating universal compassion, we create a positive feedback loop, enriching not only our own lives but the lives of others, fostering a greater harmony and balance within the interconnected web of existence. This harmony, this interconnectedness, is the very essence of spiritual growth, a path that leads not just to personal fulfillment but to a deeper understanding of our place within the grand design of the universe.

Consider the suffering in the world – the poverty, the violence, the injustice. It's easy to become overwhelmed, to feel helpless in the face of such immense challenges. Yet, the cultivation of universal compassion provides a powerful antidote to despair. It's not about solving every problem or alleviating every suffering, but about approaching each challenge with a heart filled with love and empathy. It's about offering a helping hand, a kind word, a listening ear, whenever and wherever we can.

These actions, seemingly small in isolation, possess the power to create a ripple effect of positivity, transforming not only the lives of those we directly help but also our own. The act of giving, of extending compassion, is inherently self-renewing, nourishing our souls and expanding our capacity for love. It's a testament to the interconnectedness of all things, a recognition that our own well-being is inextricably linked to the well-being of all beings.

Extending compassion to all beings is not a passive acceptance of suffering, but rather an active participation in the creation of a more compassionate world. It requires courage, determination, and a unwavering commitment to our values. It may challenge our preconceived notions and force us to confront uncomfortable truths about ourselves and the world around us. But it is through this confrontation, through this willingness to grow and evolve, that we truly unlock our potential for love and compassion.

The journey towards the immortality of the soul is not merely a pursuit of personal enlightenment, but a journey of transformation that extends beyond the individual, embracing the entire web of life. It is a journey that demands not only inner peace but also a compassionate engagement with the world around us. It is through extending love and compassion to all beings that we truly achieve a state of wholeness, a harmonious unity with the universe. This unity is the key to unlocking the potential of our souls, allowing us to transcend the limitations of the physical realm and experience a life that extends far beyond the confines of our mortal existence. This profound connection to the interconnectedness of all life is the pathway to a richer, more meaningful life, enriching the journey towards the immortality of the soul. By embracing universal compassion, we not only contribute to a more compassionate world, but we also unlock within ourselves the boundless potential for love and understanding, a path that leads to the truest form of spiritual liberation.

The Power of LovingKindness Meditation

The journey toward cultivating universal compassion, as we've discussed, is a deeply personal one, a blossoming of the heart that unfolds gradually. But this inner transformation isn't achieved in isolation; it requires dedicated practice and the conscious cultivation of loving-kindness. This is where the power of loving-kindness meditation comes into play, a potent tool for expanding our capacity for empathy and nurturing a profound connection with all beings.

Loving-kindness meditation, also known as Metta Bhavana in Pali, is a practice that involves cultivating feelings of loving-kindness, compassion, sympathetic joy, and equanimity. These four sublime states, known as the Brahma Viharas, are cornerstones of Buddhist practice, and their cultivation significantly impacts our mental, emotional, and spiritual well-being. The practice involves directing these feelings towards ourselves, loved ones, neutral individuals, and ultimately, even those we perceive as difficult or challenging. Through repeated practice, these feelings extend beyond our immediate circle, embracing a growing sphere of sentient beings, subtly reshaping our perception of the world and fostering a profound sense of interconnectedness.

Beginning the practice requires finding a quiet and comfortable space where you can sit or lie down without distractions. Focus on your breath, allowing yourself to settle into a state of calm awareness. As your body relaxes, gently bring your attention to your heart center. This doesn't need to be a literal physical sensation; it's more a focal point for your intention. Now, silently repeat a phrase or mantra associated with loving-kindness. Common phrases include

"May I be well," "May I be happy," "May I be peaceful," or "May I be free from suffering." Repeat this phrase to yourself, feeling the sincerity of each word resonating within your heart. Allow the feelings of loving-kindness to naturally arise within you. This isn't about forcing emotion; rather, it's about creating a space for it to gently bloom. Feel the warmth and kindness spreading through your being.

As you become more comfortable with directing loving-kindness towards yourself, gradually expand the circle of your compassion. Next, think of someone you love deeply – a family member, a friend, a pet. Repeat the loving-kindness phrases, directing them towards this person. Visualize them, feeling genuine affection and warmth for their well-being. Allow these feelings to flow freely, recognizing their inherent worth and deservingness of happiness and peace. Imagine them surrounded by a radiant light of love and kindness, emanating from your heart. This act of extending kindness isn't just a mental exercise; it creates a genuine energetic connection that can positively impact your relationships.

The next step is to extend loving-kindness to neutral individuals—people you encounter in your daily life but don't have a strong connection with. This could be the cashier at the grocery store, a fellow commuter, or even a stranger you see on the street. Repeat the loving-kindness phrases silently, wishing them well. This practice helps to break down barriers and cultivate a sense of connection with the world around you. The key here is to approach the practice without judgment or expectation. Simply offer your silent wishes of well-being, letting go of any personal biases or preconceived notions. This expansion of compassion helps cultivate a more inclusive and accepting worldview.

The final and most challenging step involves extending loving-kindness to those you find difficult or challenging, those who might have caused you pain or discomfort. This requires immense courage and self-awareness, as it necessitates letting go of resentment, anger, and negative emotions. Start by acknowledging their humanity. Recognize that even those who have wronged us are sentient beings experiencing their own suffering and challenges. Repeat the loving-kindness phrases, offering them your silent wishes for peace and well-being. This is not about condoning harmful actions; it's about acknowledging their suffering and offering compassion without judgment. It's a profoundly transformative practice that can significantly alleviate resentment and promote inner peace. This stage can take time and repeated practice. Don't be discouraged if you encounter resistance. Gentle persistence will yield profound results.

The key to successful loving-kindness meditation is consistency and sincerity. Even a few minutes of daily practice can bring about significant positive changes in your outlook and your relationships. The more you practice, the more natural and effortless the feelings of loving-kindness will become. These feelings won't just be confined to your meditation practice; they'll permeate your daily life, influencing your interactions with others and fostering a sense of peace and harmony within you.

To deepen your experience, incorporate visualization techniques into your meditation. Imagine a golden light emanating from your heart, enveloping yourself and those you send loving-kindness to. This visualization can enhance the feelings of warmth and connection. Experiment with different phrases and mantras that resonate with you personally. The most important aspect is that the words you use feel genuine and meaningful to you. Furthermore, the practice isn't just about repeating phrases; it's about consciously fostering a feeling of genuine compassion and kindness.

Beyond the guided meditation, consider integrating the principles of loving-kindness into your daily life. Practice acts of kindness, both big and small. Offer a helping hand to someone in need, express gratitude to those around you, and cultivate a spirit of forgiveness. These actions will reinforce the feelings cultivated during your meditation and further strengthen your capacity for compassion. Remember, the goal is not to achieve a perfect state of loving-kindness; it's about cultivating the intention and practicing regularly. Even small acts of kindness will have a ripple effect, spreading positivity to yourself and those around you, strengthening your overall energetic field.

Integrating loving-kindness meditation into a broader spiritual practice amplifies its effects. Combine it with other meditative techniques like mindfulness or breathwork. The combination of these practices creates a powerful synergy, enhancing your ability to cultivate inner peace and expand your capacity for compassion. Mindfulness helps you observe your thoughts and emotions without judgment, while breathwork helps regulate your energy and calm your nervous system. This holistic approach to spiritual practice creates a foundation for sustainable growth and transformation.

The benefits of loving-kindness meditation extend far beyond the realm of emotional well-being. Studies have shown that regular practice can reduce stress levels, improve cardiovascular health, and even boost the immune system. The cultivation of positive emotions strengthens the body's ability to heal and resist illness. This is consistent with the overall philosophy that connects spiritual well-being to physical vitality, a connection that's crucial for achieving longevity and the immortality of the soul. The cultivation of love and compassion isn't merely a spiritual exercise; it's a pathway to a healthier, happier, and more fulfilling life.

As you continue your journey towards the immortality of the soul, remember that the path isn't solely about individual enlightenment; it's about expanding your capacity for love and compassion, radiating kindness outward, and creating a ripple effect of positivity in the world. Loving-kindness meditation is a powerful tool on this journey. It's a practice that can transform not only your inner world but also your interactions with others, enriching your life and contributing to a more compassionate and harmonious world. By embracing this practice, you are not just cultivating inner peace; you are cultivating a legacy of love, a legacy that transcends the limitations of the physical realm and contributes to the overall elevation of consciousness. This higher vibrational state, nurtured through loving-kindness, is the cornerstone of a life extended beyond the physical – a life that touches the timeless essence of the soul. It is a path to a richer, more meaningful existence, one that resonates with the universe's infinite love and supports the journey towards immortality. Remember, the journey to the immortality of the soul is a journey of continuous growth and expansion, and loving-kindness meditation is a vital step on that path.

Dealing with Grief and Loss Through Meditation

Grief and loss are inevitable parts of the human experience. They are universal journeys, each unique and profoundly personal. While there's no single "right" way to grieve, meditation offers a powerful toolset to navigate these challenging emotions with grace and compassion. It's not about erasing the pain – grief is a natural and necessary process – but about creating space within yourself to experience it fully, without being overwhelmed by it. This space, cultivated through consistent meditation practice, allows you to honor your loss while simultaneously nurturing your healing.

The initial shock and disbelief that often accompany loss can be incredibly disorienting. The mind races, filled with a whirlwind of emotions: sadness, anger, guilt, regret, perhaps even numbness. In these moments, meditation acts as an anchor. Simple, mindful breathing exercises can help ground you in the present moment, providing a sense of stability amidst the chaos. Focusing on the rhythm of your breath – the gentle rise and fall of your chest or abdomen – can help to slow down the frantic pace of your thoughts and bring a sense of calm. Even just five minutes of focused breathing can significantly reduce feelings of overwhelm.

Beyond basic breathwork, guided meditations specifically designed for grief can be profoundly helpful. Many guided meditations are available online or through meditation apps, offering soothing voices and gentle prompts to guide you through the process of acknowledging and processing your emotions. These meditations often incorporate visualizations, allowing you to imagine a space of peace and healing where you can gently release your pain. Some might involve visualizing the deceased, offering a space to say goodbye or express unspoken feelings. Remember that these visualizations are tools for healing; they are not meant to replace professional help if needed.

One particularly effective technique is loving-kindness meditation, adapted for the context of grief. Instead of directing loving-kindness towards oneself and others as typically practiced, you can direct it towards the deceased, expressing feelings of love, gratitude, and forgiveness. This practice can be a powerful way to release lingering resentment or unresolved issues, allowing you to find peace and acceptance. For instance, you might silently repeat phrases like, "May you be at peace," or "May you be free from suffering," focusing on the feeling of compassion and sending those feelings towards the person you have lost.

It's crucial to remember that meditation is not a quick fix for grief. It's a practice, a journey of self-discovery and healing that unfolds over time. There will be days when you feel strong and capable, and days when the grief feels overwhelming. On those difficult days, allow yourself to feel the pain without judgment. Don't try to force yourself into a meditative state if you're not ready. Instead, simply allow yourself to be present with your emotions, acknowledging them without resistance. The very act of recognizing your feelings without trying to change them can be a powerful step towards healing.

A common challenge during grieving is the intrusion of negative self-talk. The mind might replay past events, highlighting regrets or perceived failures. This inner criticism can amplify feelings of guilt and sadness. Meditation provides tools to counteract this negativity. By observing your thoughts without judgment, you begin to create distance between yourself and your thoughts. You start to recognize them as transient phenomena, not as definitive truths about yourself. This awareness allows you to gently redirect your focus towards more positive and supportive thoughts.

For example, if you find yourself dwelling on a past argument with the deceased, you can gently acknowledge the thought, "I'm noticing I'm thinking about that argument again," and then redirect your attention to your breath or a calming visualization. This doesn't mean you're ignoring the pain, but rather, you're consciously choosing to not allow those negative thoughts to dominate your experience.

Another significant aspect of grief is the physical sensation of pain. The body often reflects emotional distress, manifesting as physical aches, tension, or fatigue. Mindfulness practices, such as body scans, can help you become more aware of these physical sensations. A body scan involves systematically bringing your attention to different parts of your body, noticing any sensations without judgment. This increased awareness can help you release physical tension associated with grief, promoting relaxation and reducing discomfort. For example, you might notice tension in your shoulders and then consciously relax them, repeating this process throughout your body.

Alongside meditation, other self-care practices are essential during the grieving process. This includes ensuring adequate sleep, maintaining a healthy diet, engaging in gentle physical activity, and seeking support from loved ones or professionals. Remember, healing from grief is not a linear process. It's a journey with ups and downs, and it's perfectly acceptable to feel a range of emotions. Meditation provides a supportive framework to navigate this journey, helping you find moments of peace and solace amidst the pain. It empowers you to connect with your inner resilience, fostering acceptance and healing over time. Be patient with yourself, and allow yourself the time and space you need to grieve.

The practice of mindfulness, a core component of meditation, also plays a vital role in navigating grief. Mindfulness encourages you to be present in the moment, without judgment or resistance. This allows you to experience the full spectrum of your emotions – the sadness, the anger, the longing – without being swept away by them. By simply acknowledging your feelings without trying to change them, you create a space for healing and self-compassion. You learn to observe your emotions as passing clouds in the sky, rather than enduring storms.

The transition from acute grief to a more integrated acceptance is a gradual process. Meditation can support this transition by helping you develop a sense of perspective. As you cultivate a deeper awareness of your inner world, you begin to see your experiences in a broader context. You may realize that even the deepest pain is temporary, that life is a cycle of change, and that you possess the inner strength to navigate even the most challenging circumstances.

Integrating meditation into your daily routine, even for short periods, can be a profoundly transformative practice during grieving. Consider making it a part of your morning or evening routine, or incorporating short mindfulness breaks throughout your day. These regular practices can help you create a sense of stability and inner peace, even amidst emotional turmoil.

Moreover, the healing power of meditation extends beyond the individual. It can also strengthen your relationships with others who are also grieving. Sharing your meditation practice with loved ones can create a sense of shared connection and mutual support. This could involve attending a meditation group together, practicing mindfulness together, or simply sharing your experiences with each other. This shared journey can foster a deeper understanding and strengthen bonds during a challenging time. The supportive energy created through shared meditation can be profoundly healing.

Ultimately, meditation is a tool for self-empowerment in the face of loss. It helps you access your inner resources, fostering resilience, self-compassion, and a sense of peace. It's a journey of self-discovery, allowing you to connect with your deepest self and find strength within to navigate the complexities of grief and emerge stronger on the other side. Remember that seeking professional help from a therapist or counselor is perfectly acceptable and often beneficial in conjunction with meditation practices. The combination of professional guidance and personal mindfulness can offer a powerful path towards healing and lasting peace. Allow yourself the time and compassion you deserve during this journey.

Managing Stress and Anxiety Through Mindfulness

Building upon the foundation of inner peace cultivated through navigating grief and loss, we now turn our attention to another pervasive challenge of modern life: stress and anxiety. These are not merely inconveniences; they are significant impediments to spiritual growth and the longevity we seek. Chronic stress wreaks havoc on the body and mind, impacting everything from our immune system to our emotional resilience. However, the principles of mindfulness, deeply intertwined with meditation, provide potent antidotes to these pervasive modern ailments.

The very nature of stress lies in the constant pull between our present moment and our anxieties about the future, or regrets about the past. Mindfulness, at its core, is the art of returning to the present. It's about gently redirecting our attention from the racing thoughts, the worries, and the anxieties that fuel stress and anxiety, and anchoring it in the here and now. This is not about ignoring our problems; rather, it's about creating space between ourselves and those problems, observing them without judgment, and responding rather than reacting.

One of the most accessible mindfulness techniques for stress reduction is the practice of mindful breathing. Find a comfortable position, whether sitting or lying down. Close your eyes gently, and bring your attention to the sensation of your breath entering and leaving your body. Notice the rise and fall of your chest or abdomen. Don't try to control your breath; simply observe it. If your mind wanders—and it will—gently guide it back to the sensation of your breath. This simple act of focusing on the present moment, on the rhythm of your breath, can have a profound calming effect on your nervous system.

Expand this practice by incorporating body scans. Once you've established a comfortable rhythm of mindful breathing, begin to bring your attention to different parts of your body. Start with your toes, noticing any sensations – tingling, warmth, pressure, or coolness. Move slowly upwards, through your feet, ankles, calves, and so on, until you've scanned your entire body. Again, the key is to observe without judgment, simply acknowledging the sensations without trying to change them. This practice not only relaxes the body, but also cultivates a deeper awareness of your physical self, grounding you in the present moment.

Mindful walking is another effective technique. Instead of rushing through your day, take time for a mindful walk. Pay attention to the sensation of your feet making contact with the ground, the rhythm of your steps, the movement of your body. Notice the sounds around you – the rustling of leaves, the chirping of birds, the gentle breeze. Observe the sights – the colors, the shapes, the textures. Engage all your senses, fully present in each step. This simple act transforms a mundane activity into a meditative practice, calming the mind and connecting you with the natural world.

Beyond these foundational practices, we can incorporate mindfulness into our daily routines. Eating mindfully, for instance, involves savoring each bite, paying attention to the tastes, textures, and aromas of your food. Instead of rushing through meals, take the time to truly appreciate the nourishment you're receiving. Similarly, engage in mindful listening when interacting with others. Focus on what they are saying, paying attention not only to their words but also to their tone and body language. This creates a deeper connection, reduces misunderstandings, and fosters a sense of peace and understanding.

The power of mindfulness extends to our thoughts and emotions as well. When stressful or anxious thoughts arise, don't fight them or try to suppress them. Instead, acknowledge them, observe them, and let them pass. Think of your mind as a clear sky, and your thoughts as clouds drifting by. They may appear and disappear, but the sky remains clear and unperturbed. This detached observation prevents you from becoming overwhelmed by your thoughts and emotions.

Furthermore, cultivate self-compassion. Be kind and understanding towards yourself, particularly during times of stress and anxiety. Treat yourself with the same compassion and understanding you would offer a dear friend facing similar challenges. Remind yourself that it's okay to feel stressed or anxious; it's a normal part of the human experience. However, it's not necessary to be controlled *by* those feelings. Mindfulness provides the tools to navigate these emotions with grace and equanimity.

The practice of loving-kindness meditation can further enhance your resilience to stress. This involves cultivating feelings of love and compassion, not only for yourself but also for others. Start by directing loving-kindness towards yourself, wishing yourself well-being and happiness. Then extend these feelings to loved ones, friends, acquaintances, and eventually even to those you find difficult to love. This practice cultivates a sense of interconnectedness and compassion, reducing feelings of isolation and fostering inner peace.

Maintaining a regular meditation practice is crucial for effectively managing stress and anxiety. Even short, daily sessions of 10-15 minutes can make a significant difference. Consistency is key; make meditation a non-negotiable part of your daily routine, like brushing your teeth or having your morning coffee. This consistent practice trains your mind to remain calm and centered in the face of adversity.

Integrating mindfulness into your daily life is a continuous process, a journey of self-discovery. There will be days when your practice feels effortless, and there will be days when it feels challenging. Be patient with yourself, celebrate your successes, and learn from your setbacks. Remember that mindfulness is not about achieving perfection; it's about cultivating a consistent and compassionate awareness of the present moment.

Incorporating mindfulness into our lives isn't simply a matter of techniques; it's a shift in perspective. It's about viewing challenges not as threats but as opportunities for growth and learning. It's about understanding that the storms of life are transient; the inner calm cultivated through meditation endures. This is the essence of navigating life's challenges with grace: accepting what we cannot change, changing what we can, and having the wisdom to know the difference. This wisdom, in turn, directly contributes to a longer, healthier, and more spiritually fulfilling life, extending the very essence of our being beyond the limitations of the physical body. The journey towards the immortality of the soul is paved with mindful moments, each one bringing us closer to a state of enduring peace and serenity. And this peace, this inner tranquility, is the ultimate antidote to the stresses and anxieties that plague modern life. The journey is not about eliminating stress entirely, but about cultivating the inner strength and resilience to meet life's challenges with equanimity and compassion, allowing us to live a richer, fuller, and more meaningful existence. This resilience, forged in the crucible of mindful practice, allows us to navigate not only the present challenges but to face the future with unwavering confidence and a deep sense of inner peace. The ultimate goal is not the eradication of stress but its transformation into a catalyst for growth and spiritual evolution. Each stressful encounter becomes an opportunity to deepen our practice, to refine our ability to respond with wisdom and compassion, ultimately leading to a more harmonious relationship with ourselves and the world around us. This harmonious relationship, nurtured through consistent mindfulness, is the cornerstone of a long and spiritually meaningful life, a testament to the transformative power of mindful living and a vital step towards the immortality of the soul.

Finding Strength and Resilience in Difficult Times

Building upon the foundation of inner peace cultivated through mindful engagement with life's inevitable difficulties, we now delve deeper into the practical application of meditation for fostering inner strength and resilience. The ability to navigate challenges with grace isn't merely a passive acceptance; it's an active cultivation of inner resources that allow us to not only endure, but to thrive, even amidst adversity. This resilience, deeply rooted in the consistent practice of meditation, becomes a powerful tool for self-empowerment, transforming obstacles into opportunities for growth and spiritual evolution.

One of the key aspects of building resilience lies in understanding the nature of suffering. We often perceive challenges as external threats, as forces outside our control that inflict pain and hardship upon us. However, a deeper understanding reveals that suffering is not inherent in the event itself, but rather in our interpretation of it. It is our reaction, our attachment to a particular outcome, that creates the suffering. Meditation helps us to detach from these reactive patterns, allowing us to observe our thoughts and emotions without judgment, creating a space between stimulus and response. This space, this pause, is where the power of resilience emerges.

Consider the example of a significant loss – the death of a loved one, a failed business venture, or a broken relationship. Initially, the pain can be overwhelming, leaving us feeling helpless and adrift. However, through consistent meditation, we gradually cultivate the ability to observe these emotions without being consumed by them. We recognize that grief, sorrow, and disappointment are natural responses to loss, but they are not our identity. They are temporary states, passing clouds in the ever-changing sky of our consciousness. By practicing mindful awareness, we create space around these emotions, allowing them to arise and pass without clinging to them. This detached awareness doesn't negate the pain; rather, it softens its intensity and allows us to find a place of acceptance and even peace within the turmoil.

This ability to observe without judgment extends beyond emotional challenges. Physical ailments, financial difficulties, and relationship conflicts can all be navigated with greater ease and grace through the practice of mindful meditation. When faced with a stressful situation, the tendency is to react instinctively, often with fear, anger, or anxiety. However, by pausing, taking a few deep breaths, and focusing on the present moment, we can disrupt this reactive pattern and create space for a more considered response. This conscious pause allows us to access our inner wisdom, enabling us to make choices that align with our values and long-term well-being. This conscious response, grounded in mindfulness, is the hallmark of true resilience.

Moreover, meditation equips us with the tools to cultivate inner strength – a sense of self-assurance and unwavering resolve that allows us to face adversity with courage and determination. This inner strength isn't about suppressing our emotions or pretending that everything is okay. It's about recognizing our vulnerability, accepting our imperfections, and drawing upon our inner reserves of compassion, empathy, and strength to meet whatever life throws our way. It's the realization that we are not defined by our challenges, but by our response to them.

Developing this inner strength is a gradual process, nurtured by consistent meditation practice. Regular meditation cultivates a deeper connection with our inner self, allowing us to access a reservoir of inner peace and stability that serves as a constant anchor amidst the storms of life. Through meditation, we come to understand that we are not our thoughts or emotions; we are the awareness that observes them. This awareness, this consciousness, is the foundation of our resilience.

The practice of self-compassion is also essential in building resilience. We are often our own harshest critics, judging ourselves harshly for perceived failures and shortcomings. This self-criticism, this inner negativity, only exacerbates stress and anxiety, weakening our ability to cope with challenges. Meditation helps us cultivate self-compassion, allowing us to treat ourselves with the same kindness and understanding that we would offer a friend in need. This involves acknowledging our imperfections, accepting our vulnerabilities, and offering ourselves the support and encouragement we need to overcome difficulties.

This practice of self-compassion extends to our interactions with others. When faced with challenging relationships, we often react defensively, adding fuel to the fire of conflict. However, through meditation, we develop the ability to approach these situations with greater empathy and understanding. We see the other person's perspective, recognizing that their actions may stem from their own pain and suffering. This empathetic understanding allows us to respond with compassion rather than judgment, creating a space for healing and reconciliation.

Furthermore, cultivating gratitude plays a pivotal role in building resilience. When we focus on what we lack, we perpetuate feelings of scarcity and dissatisfaction. However, when we cultivate an attitude of gratitude, focusing on the good things in our lives, we shift our perspective, creating a more positive and resilient mindset. This practice of gratitude doesn't ignore the challenges we face, but rather places them in a broader context of appreciation for the blessings we already possess. Through meditation, we learn to recognize and cherish these blessings, fostering a sense of contentment and inner peace that strengthens our ability to navigate life's inevitable ups and downs.

Finally, building resilience involves cultivating a sense of purpose and meaning in our lives. When we feel a deep connection to something larger than ourselves, whether it's our family, our community, or a spiritual practice, we find a source of strength and motivation that helps us overcome obstacles. This sense of purpose anchors us, giving us the resilience to persevere even when the going gets tough. Meditation facilitates this connection by deepening our self-awareness and our understanding of our place in the larger scheme of things. It helps us connect with our values, clarifying our intentions and inspiring action aligned with a greater purpose. This conscious alignment with our values and our purpose enhances resilience, providing a framework for decision-making and action even during stressful times.

In conclusion, the journey towards building inner strength and resilience is a continuous process, a journey of self-discovery and growth fueled by consistent meditation practice. It's not about eliminating challenges, but about cultivating the inner resources to navigate them with grace, wisdom, and compassion. Through the cultivation of mindful awareness, self-compassion, gratitude, and a sense of purpose, we develop the inner strength to not only endure adversity but to emerge from it transformed, strengthened, and deeply connected to our true selves—a testament to the transformative power of meditation and a crucial step on the path towards the immortality of the soul. This resilience, nurtured through consistent mindful practice, is the cornerstone of a long, fulfilling, and spiritually meaningful life, a life that transcends the limitations of the physical realm and extends towards the boundless horizons of the spirit. The ability to face life's trials with grace is not simply about surviving; it is about thriving, about transforming challenges into opportunities for profound personal growth and spiritual evolution. It is about embracing the journey, accepting the lessons, and emerging stronger, wiser, and more deeply connected to the essence of our being.

Letting Go of Control and Embracing Acceptance

The journey towards spiritual enlightenment, as we've explored, is paved with both moments of profound peace and periods of intense challenge. While cultivating inner strength and resilience is paramount, true mastery lies in understanding when to exert effort and when to gracefully surrender to the unfolding of life. This is the essence of letting go of control and embracing acceptance—a powerful tool not for passivity, but for navigating life's complexities with wisdom and equanimity.

Many of us are conditioned to believe that control equals security. We strive to meticulously plan our lives, seeking to anticipate and manage every potential obstacle. While a degree of planning and preparedness is undoubtedly beneficial, the relentless pursuit of control often leads to frustration, anxiety, and a sense of being overwhelmed. Life, in its inherent unpredictability, frequently throws curveballs, rendering our meticulously crafted plans irrelevant. This is not a failure; it is simply the nature of existence. The universe, in its infinite wisdom, unfolds in ways often beyond our comprehension, and clinging to the illusion of complete control only serves to amplify our suffering.

The path to acceptance begins with self-awareness. Through consistent meditation practice, we become increasingly attuned to our thoughts, emotions, and reactions. We begin to observe the patterns that govern our behavior, noticing how we react to setbacks and unexpected events. This self-observation is crucial, as it allows us to identify the grip we hold on control and to understand the limitations of our ability to predict and manipulate outcomes. The more we practice mindful awareness, the more we recognize that our attachment to control stems from fear—fear of the unknown, fear of failure, fear of loss.

Letting go of control isn't about relinquishing responsibility. It's about shifting our perspective from a place of rigid control to one of flexible adaptation. It's about accepting that some things are simply beyond our direct influence, and choosing to respond to life's challenges with grace rather than resistance. This doesn't mean passivity; it means responding with wisdom, discernment, and a willingness to adapt to the changing circumstances. It means recognizing that even setbacks can be valuable learning experiences, guiding us towards growth and a deeper understanding of ourselves and the world around us.

This process often requires us to confront our ego, that part of ourselves that clings to the illusion of control and craves validation. The ego thrives on the illusion of separateness, believing it can dictate the course of events. However, letting go of control invites us to surrender to a larger, interconnected reality, where we are but a small part of a vast and intricate web of existence. This surrender is not a sign of weakness, but a testament to our willingness to embrace our true nature—a part of something far greater than ourselves.

Consider the analogy of a river flowing towards the ocean. The river encounters countless obstacles—rocks, rapids, waterfalls—yet it continues its journey, adapting its course to navigate these challenges. It doesn't resist the obstacles; it integrates them into its flow. Similarly, in life, we encounter numerous obstacles, both internal and external. The path to acceptance lies in learning to navigate these challenges with the same fluidity and grace as the river, adapting our course as needed while maintaining our overall direction.

This process of letting go often requires us to confront our limiting beliefs. These are the deeply ingrained patterns of thought that perpetuate our fear and resistance to change. Through meditation and self-reflection, we can identify these beliefs and begin to challenge their validity. We can replace them with empowering beliefs that support our growth and facilitate our ability to accept the unpredictable nature of life. This is a gradual process, requiring patience, self-compassion, and a willingness to let go of outdated and unhelpful patterns of thinking.

Embracing acceptance also involves cultivating a deep sense of trust in the universe. This trust arises from a growing understanding that everything happens for a reason, even if that reason is not immediately apparent. It is a recognition that life's challenges, though often painful, serve a purpose —to teach us valuable lessons, to strengthen our resilience, and to guide us towards our highest potential. Trusting in this process doesn't negate the challenges; it allows us to approach them with a different perspective, one of faith and hope rather than fear and resistance.

This trust is nurtured through regular meditation practice, allowing us to connect with a deeper sense of peace and understanding. Meditation allows us to quiet the incessant chatter of the mind, creating space for intuition and insight to emerge. It helps us to connect with our inner wisdom, which knows that everything unfolds according to a divine plan, even if we cannot fully grasp it in the present moment. This faith empowers us to accept the unknown with courage and serenity.

Furthermore, acceptance necessitates cultivating compassion, not only for ourselves but also for others. When we encounter difficulties, it's easy to become self-critical, to dwell on our perceived failures and shortcomings. However, self-compassion is essential. We must treat ourselves with the same kindness and understanding that we would offer a close friend facing similar challenges. This allows us to navigate difficult times with greater ease and reduces the suffering often associated with feelings of self-blame and inadequacy. Extending this compassion to others enhances our understanding and empathy, strengthening our ability to navigate the complexities of human interaction with greater grace.

The path to letting go of control and embracing acceptance is not a destination but a continuous journey. It requires ongoing effort, self-awareness, and a commitment to consistent meditation practice. It's a process of continual learning and growth, where each challenge presents an opportunity to deepen our understanding of ourselves and the world around us. It is through this process of surrender and acceptance that we truly begin to navigate life's challenges with grace, transforming adversity into opportunities for profound spiritual growth and evolving towards a deeper connection with our true selves, ultimately paving the way for the immortality of the soul.

This journey requires courage, a willingness to step outside of our comfort zones, and to embrace the unknown. It's about relinquishing the illusion of control and trusting in the natural flow of life. It's about acknowledging our limitations while celebrating our strengths. It's about embracing the paradox of surrender and action, recognizing that we can both act with intention and accept the unpredictable nature of outcomes. This paradoxical approach is essential for navigating life's complexities with grace, allowing us to maintain a sense of purpose and direction while remaining open to the unexpected twists and turns of the journey.

Consider the challenges you've faced in the past. Reflect on how you responded to them. Did you cling to control, striving to dictate outcomes? Or did you find a way to adapt, to find flexibility in the face of unexpected events? By reflecting on past experiences, we can gain valuable insights into our patterns of behavior and begin to identify areas where we can cultivate greater acceptance. This self-reflection is a vital component of the journey towards letting go, allowing us to learn from our past experiences and to cultivate greater wisdom in our approach to future challenges.

The practice of meditation plays a pivotal role in this process. By regularly engaging in meditation, we train our minds to focus on the present moment, allowing us to release the grip of past regrets and future anxieties. We develop a greater capacity for self-awareness, allowing us to observe our thoughts and emotions without judgment. This increased self-awareness is essential for identifying and releasing the patterns of thought and behavior that perpetuate our clinging to control. The tranquility cultivated through meditation strengthens our ability to accept the unfolding of life with grace and equanimity.

Ultimately, letting go of control and embracing acceptance is a pathway to profound freedom. It is through this surrender that we unlock the potential for genuine peace, allowing us to experience life with a greater sense of joy and appreciation. It is not about resignation but about finding a deeper understanding of our place within the vast and intricate tapestry of existence. It is about releasing the burden of unnecessary control and embracing the flow of life with open hearts and minds, confident in the knowledge that we are guided by a force far greater than ourselves, a force that leads us ultimately towards the immortality of the soul. The acceptance of this journey, the acceptance of the

unpredictable, is the ultimate key to unlocking the limitless
potential within us all.

Transforming Suffering into Wisdom

The path to spiritual enlightenment, as we've touched upon, isn't a smooth, uninterrupted ascent. It's a journey marked by both luminous peaks of joy and profound valleys of suffering. While the previous chapter emphasized the importance of graceful surrender and acceptance, this section delves into the transformative power of adversity itself. It's not about avoiding hardship, for that's an impossible task; rather, it's about harnessing the potential for wisdom embedded within every challenge, every setback, every seemingly insurmountable obstacle.

Suffering, in its raw and unfiltered form, is often perceived as an enemy, something to be avoided, suppressed, or escaped. We build walls around our hearts, erecting defenses against pain and disappointment, believing that if we can just maintain a state of perpetual comfort, we'll somehow find lasting peace. But true peace, the kind that resonates deep within the soul and anchors us to a higher truth, isn't found in the absence of suffering; it's found in our response to it. It's in the crucible of difficult experiences that the purest gold of wisdom is forged.

Consider the metaphor of the blacksmith and the ore. Raw ore, in its unrefined state, is essentially worthless. But through intense heat and skillful manipulation, the blacksmith transforms it into something beautiful, strong, and profoundly useful. Similarly, life's challenges—the emotional blows, the setbacks, the losses—are the raw ore of our spiritual journey. They may feel harsh and unpleasant at the time, but they contain the potential for incredible transformation. It's through the "fire" of adversity that we are refined, strengthened, and ultimately, elevated.

This transformative process isn't passive; it requires conscious engagement. It requires us to confront our suffering, not to shy away from it, but to meet it head-on with courage, compassion, and a willingness to learn. This isn't about finding some simplistic, feel-good solution to every problem. Instead, it's about cultivating a deep inner resilience, a capacity to navigate the inevitable storms of life with grace, strength, and a profound understanding that even the darkest nights eventually yield to the dawn.

One crucial element in this process is cultivating self-compassion. During times of hardship, it's easy to fall into self-criticism, to berate ourselves for our perceived failures or shortcomings. We may replay past events in our minds, analyzing every mistake, every missed opportunity, reinforcing feelings of guilt, shame, and inadequacy. But this self-flagellation only serves to amplify the suffering. Self-compassion, on the other hand, offers a different perspective. It involves treating ourselves with the same kindness and understanding that we would extend to a dear friend facing similar struggles.

It acknowledges that we are all imperfect, that we are all capable of making mistakes, and that these experiences, while painful, are a natural part of the human journey. Instead of focusing on what went wrong, self-compassion allows us to focus on what we can learn from the experience, to acknowledge our pain without judgment, and to gently guide ourselves towards healing and growth. This compassionate self-reflection is essential for transforming suffering into wisdom.

Another key aspect of this transformation is the development of a broader perspective. When we're immersed in suffering, our focus tends to narrow, fixating on our immediate pain and discomfort. We lose sight of the bigger picture, forgetting that our lives are part of a larger context, embedded within a universe that operates according to its own laws and rhythms. Developing a broader perspective involves cultivating a sense of detachment from our ego-centric viewpoint, allowing us to see our challenges as opportunities for growth, rather than as personal failures or punishments.

This isn't to say that we should diminish the significance of our suffering; rather, it's about shifting our perspective, broadening our understanding of the interconnectedness of all things. Recognizing that our struggles are part of a larger tapestry of experience—a tapestry woven with threads of joy and sorrow, light and darkness—allows us to find meaning and purpose even in the midst of pain. This broader perspective fosters resilience, fostering a belief in our ability to persevere and emerge stronger from even the most challenging of circumstances.

Furthermore, the process of transforming suffering into wisdom involves cultivating gratitude. This may seem counterintuitive—how can we be grateful in the midst of hardship?—but gratitude acts as a powerful antidote to negativity and despair. When we focus on what we have, rather than what we lack, we shift our attention away from our pain and towards the blessings in our lives. This doesn't mean ignoring the challenges we face; rather, it's about recognizing the presence of goodness alongside the darkness, cultivating an attitude of appreciation for the gifts we've been given, even in the face of adversity.

Gratitude fosters a sense of resilience. It reminds us that we possess inner strength, resources, and support, even when our circumstances feel overwhelming. It allows us to see the light amidst the darkness, strengthening our faith in our ability to overcome obstacles and find meaning in our experiences. This practice of gratitude, consistently cultivated, shifts our perspective from one of scarcity and lack to one of abundance and possibility, transforming the way we experience and respond to suffering.

Finally, the transformation of suffering into wisdom is inextricably linked to our spiritual growth. It's through confronting our challenges that we uncover our deepest limitations and fears, pushing us to confront our deepest vulnerabilities. This process, while painful, opens us to a deeper level of self-awareness, pushing us towards greater levels of self-understanding, compassion, and empathy. By facing our suffering head-on, we break down the barriers that separate us from our true selves, revealing the strength, resilience, and wisdom that lie dormant within. It's within the crucible of these trials that we ultimately discover our deepest spiritual potential.

Consider the examples of individuals who have overcome immense hardship: Nelson Mandela, imprisoned for decades, emerged as a global symbol of hope and forgiveness; Mother Teresa, witnessing immense poverty and suffering, dedicated her life to serving the poorest of the poor; individuals who have lost loved ones to tragedy, finding ways to channel their grief into acts of service and support for others. These stories powerfully illustrate the transformative power of suffering, highlighting how profound adversity can lead to unparalleled spiritual growth and inspire profound acts of compassion and service to the world.

It's not about romanticizing suffering, but about recognizing its inherent potential for growth and transformation. It's about recognizing the profound wisdom that can be gleaned from navigating life's trials, transforming them from sources of despair into opportunities for profound self-discovery and spiritual evolution. The lessons learned in these dark chapters of our lives are often the most valuable, shaping our character, strengthening our resolve, and ultimately, leading us towards a deeper understanding of ourselves and our place within the grand scheme of existence. These transformative experiences are crucial stepping stones on the path toward the immortality of the soul. The ability to transform suffering into wisdom is a hallmark of spiritual maturity, a testament to our resilience and our capacity for growth, guiding us closer to the profound peace and enlightenment we all seek. It's through this acceptance and transformation that we truly begin to embrace the limitless possibilities that lie within. The acceptance of this ongoing process, the embracing of the unpredictable, is the ultimate key to unlocking the limitless potential within us all, leading to a richer, deeper, and more fulfilling connection with the divine, ultimately culminating in the immortality of the soul.

Connecting with Your Higher Self

Connecting with your Higher Self is a journey of profound self-discovery, a pilgrimage into the depths of your being to uncover the boundless wisdom and potential residing within. It's not about reaching some distant, ethereal entity; rather, it's about recognizing and integrating the inherent divinity already present within you. This connection isn't a mystical feat reserved for a select few; it's an inherent capacity available to everyone willing to embark on the path of self-reflection and mindful exploration.

The concept of a Higher Self often evokes images of a celestial being or a separate spiritual entity. However, a more accurate understanding positions the Higher Self as the truest essence of your being, the core of your consciousness unburdened by the limitations of ego, fear, and societal conditioning. It's the part of you that knows your deepest desires, your truest purpose, and the path that leads you to a life of profound meaning and fulfillment. Imagine it as the silent wisdom whispering beneath the noise of your daily thoughts and anxieties.

Connecting with your Higher Self isn't about silencing the chattering mind entirely. Instead, it's about learning to navigate the stream of consciousness, to observe your thoughts and emotions without judgment, allowing them to flow naturally without clinging to them. This process, often described as witnessing, allows the quiet voice of your Higher Self to emerge from the background noise. It's in these moments of quiet observation that you begin to access a deeper wellspring of creativity, intuition, and inner guidance.

One of the most effective pathways to connecting with your Higher Self is through dedicated meditation practices. Regular meditation allows you to cultivate a space of stillness within, a sanctuary where the incessant chatter of the ego fades, allowing the deeper wisdom of your Higher Self to emerge. Start with short, focused meditation sessions, gradually increasing the duration as you become more comfortable. Find a quiet space where you won't be disturbed, and focus on your breath, allowing the rhythm of your inhalations and exhalations to anchor you in the present moment.

As you deepen your meditation practice, you'll notice shifts in your awareness. You may experience moments of clarity and insight, a sense of profound peace and connection. These moments are glimpses into the realm of your Higher Self, moments where you tap into your innate wisdom and potential. Don't strive to force these moments; instead, cultivate a receptive attitude, allowing them to unfold organically in their own time.

Beyond formal meditation, there are numerous other ways to connect with your Higher Self. Spending time in nature can be deeply transformative. The quiet solitude of a forest, the vast expanse of the ocean, or the serene beauty of a mountain vista can all help to quiet the mind and open you to a deeper connection with yourself and the universe. Engaging in creative activities like painting, writing, music, or dance can also unlock the creative wellspring of your Higher Self, allowing you to express your inner world through outward expression.

Journaling can become a powerful tool in this process. Allow yourself to write freely, expressing whatever comes to mind without judgment or censorship. This can help to uncover hidden thoughts and beliefs that might be hindering your connection with your Higher Self. As you write, pay attention to recurring themes, intuitive insights, or feelings that emerge. These often represent valuable clues from your Higher Self, offering guidance and direction.

Actively seeking out experiences that resonate deeply with your soul is another crucial aspect of this journey. This might involve traveling to places that call to you, engaging in activities that inspire you, or connecting with people who uplift and support your growth. These experiences can help to illuminate your path, revealing your deepest passions and purpose.

Introspection plays a vital role in this process. Regularly take time for self-reflection, considering your values, beliefs, and aspirations. Ask yourself profound questions about your life, your purpose, and your place in the world. These introspective exercises can help to clarify your path and reveal the guidance offered by your Higher Self.

Connecting with your Higher Self is not a destination but a journey. It's a continuous process of self-discovery and unfolding. As you deepen your connection, you'll experience a growing sense of clarity, purpose, and self-acceptance. You'll find that life's challenges become less daunting, and your ability to navigate them with grace and resilience increases significantly.

The path to connecting with your Higher Self is often paved with unexpected twists and turns. There will be moments of doubt and uncertainty, times when the path seems unclear. These are natural parts of the process. Remember to be patient with yourself, trusting that the journey itself is a significant part of the unfolding. The challenges you encounter serve as opportunities for growth, refining your understanding of yourself and your path.

As you cultivate a deeper connection with your Higher Self, you'll find a growing sense of inner peace and contentment. You'll recognize that true happiness is not found in external achievements or material possessions but in the profound connection with your own inner essence. This deep sense of peace transcends external circumstances, offering resilience and a sense of groundedness amidst life's uncertainties.

Finding meaning and purpose in life is a fundamental human aspiration. The connection with your Higher Self provides a powerful compass, guiding you toward a life aligned with your deepest values and passions. It helps you to identify your unique talents and gifts, enabling you to contribute meaningfully to the world and to live a life of authenticity and fulfillment. This purpose isn't something imposed from the outside; rather, it's an intrinsic part of your essence, waiting to be discovered.

Your Higher Self often speaks to you in subtle ways, through intuition, inspiration, and synchronicities. Pay attention to recurring thoughts, feelings, or experiences that seem to be calling you in a particular direction. These subtle nudges are messages from your Higher Self, gently guiding you towards a life of greater purpose and fulfillment. Learning to recognize these subtle cues is crucial in navigating the path with grace and confidence.

The connection with your Higher Self is also deeply connected to the concept of intuition. As you deepen your practice, your intuition will become stronger, more reliable, and more readily available. This intuitive guidance helps you to make decisions aligned with your authentic self, fostering a sense of clarity and confidence in your choices. It's about learning to trust your inner voice, even when the external world may seem to offer contradictory guidance.

One of the most significant benefits of connecting with your Higher Self is the development of unconditional self-love. This is not about self-indulgence or narcissism; it's about accepting yourself completely, flaws and all, recognizing your inherent worthiness and value. This self-acceptance allows you to approach life's challenges with greater resilience and compassion, both towards yourself and others.

The journey to connecting with your Higher Self is a lifelong process of growth, learning, and self-discovery. There is no single endpoint; it's a continuous evolution, a constant unfolding of your potential. Embrace the process, trusting the journey, and allow yourself to be transformed by the profound wisdom residing within. The path is uniquely yours, and as you walk it with openness and intention, the wisdom of your Higher Self will illuminate your way, leading you to a life of profound meaning, purpose, and lasting fulfillment. This journey is not just about achieving immortality of the soul, but about experiencing the immortality of your spirit here, in this life, enriching every moment with a deeper connection to the profound wisdom within.

Understanding the Nature of Consciousness and Existence

The journey towards liberation and the immortality of the soul necessitates a deep understanding of the nature of consciousness and existence itself. We've explored the connection to the Higher Self, the wellspring of wisdom and potential within, but to truly grasp the implications of this connection, we must delve into the fundamental fabric of reality. What is consciousness? Is it solely a product of the brain, a fleeting spark extinguished with the death of the physical body? Or is it something far more profound, a timeless essence existing beyond the confines of our physical form?

Many spiritual traditions propose that consciousness is not limited to the brain. Instead, it's a universal energy, a fundamental aspect of the cosmos, pervading all things. From the smallest subatomic particle to the largest galaxy, this consciousness permeates existence, connecting everything in an intricate web of interconnectedness. Our individual consciousness, then, is not separate from this universal consciousness, but rather a unique expression, a wave in the ocean of cosmic awareness. This perspective offers a radical shift in our understanding of ourselves and our place in the universe. We are not isolated entities, but integral parts of a vast, interconnected whole.

This understanding has profound implications for our concept of existence. If consciousness is not limited to the brain, then the death of the physical body does not necessarily equate to the annihilation of consciousness. Instead, it may represent a transition, a shift in state, a movement from one level of existence to another. This possibility has fueled countless spiritual beliefs and philosophical inquiries throughout history. The idea of an afterlife, a realm beyond the physical, resonates with many because it offers a sense of continuity, a promise that our essence persists beyond the limitations of our physical form.

The concept of "immortality of the soul" often evokes images of a celestial afterlife, a heaven or paradise where the righteous are rewarded with eternal bliss. While such imagery can be comforting and inspirational, it's important to consider a broader, more nuanced understanding of this concept. Immortality, in this context, doesn't necessarily refer to an eternal existence in a specific location or a static state of being. Instead, it speaks to the enduring nature of consciousness itself, its capacity to transcend the limitations of time and space. Our true essence, the soul, is not bound by the physical constraints of the body; it exists beyond the limitations of birth and death.

Consider the analogy of a river. The river flows continuously, its waters ever-changing, yet the river itself remains. Individual droplets of water may enter and exit, yet the river's essence persists. Similarly, our physical bodies are like the individual droplets, temporary vessels for the flow of consciousness. The body ages, decays, and eventually dissolves, but the underlying consciousness, the essence of the soul, continues its flow, transforming, evolving, but never truly ceasing to exist.

This understanding requires a shift in perspective. We must move beyond a purely materialistic worldview, one that reduces existence to mere physical phenomena. Instead, we need to embrace a more holistic perspective that acknowledges the existence of non-physical realities, realms of energy and consciousness that extend beyond our immediate sensory perception. This is not a blind leap of faith, but rather a reasoned exploration of the mysteries of existence.

Through the practice of deep meditation, we can begin to experience this deeper reality. As we quiet the mind and still the body, we can access states of consciousness that transcend our ordinary waking awareness. These states often reveal profound insights into the interconnectedness of all things, the boundless nature of consciousness, and the enduring essence of the soul. Meditation is not merely a relaxation technique; it's a powerful tool for expanding our awareness and connecting with the deeper levels of our being.

The exploration of consciousness and existence is not limited to intellectual pursuits; it is deeply experiential. Through practices such as meditation, mindfulness, and contemplative prayer, we can cultivate a deeper understanding of our own inner nature and our connection to the universe. The goal is not simply to gather information or accumulate knowledge, but to transform our understanding into lived experience. This transformation occurs as we embody the principles we learn, integrating them into our daily lives, and allowing them to shape our thoughts, feelings, and actions.

The path to liberation and the immortality of the soul is a path of self-discovery, a journey into the depths of our being. It is a process of uncovering the inherent wisdom and potential that resides within each of us. This process involves letting go of limiting beliefs and attachments that bind us to a sense of separateness and limitation. It's about cultivating a sense of compassion, understanding, and connection with all beings, recognizing our shared essence as expressions of the same universal consciousness.

The physical body is a temporary vessel, a vehicle for our journey through this lifetime. While we cherish and care for our physical well-being, we must also recognize its limitations. The pursuit of immortality, therefore, is not about prolonging the life of the physical body indefinitely, but about cultivating the immortality of our consciousness, our soul. This involves nourishing and strengthening our inner essence, nurturing our spiritual growth, and expanding our awareness beyond the confines of our physical existence.

Throughout history, spiritual traditions across the globe have offered various techniques and practices to foster this inner growth and expand awareness. From ancient yogic practices to modern mindfulness techniques, these methods offer paths toward connecting with the deeper dimensions of our being, allowing us to experience the boundless nature of consciousness and cultivate a sense of inner peace and liberation. These practices are not merely theoretical; they are practical tools that allow us to experience directly the truths they convey.

The understanding of consciousness and existence profoundly impacts our approach to life. When we see ourselves as limited beings, confined to a single life span, we may become preoccupied with accumulating material possessions, seeking fleeting pleasures, and fearing death. However, when we recognize the timeless essence of our soul, the boundless nature of consciousness, our perspective shifts. We become less attached to the transient aspects of life and more focused on cultivating inner peace, compassion, and meaningful connections with others.

The fear of death often stems from a lack of understanding of our true nature. We identify so strongly with our physical bodies that we fear their demise as the end of our existence. However, as we deepen our understanding of consciousness and its relationship to the physical body, the fear of death begins to diminish. Death is not an ending, but a transition, a passage from one state of being to another. The essence of our being continues, even beyond the limitations of our physical form.

This understanding leads to a greater appreciation for the present moment. Life is not a rehearsal for some future existence; it is a precious gift, a unique opportunity to express our unique essence and contribute to the world around us. Each moment becomes a sacred opportunity for growth, learning, and connection. We live more fully, more consciously, with a deep appreciation for the beauty and wonder of life.

The path to liberation and the immortality of the soul is not a solitary journey. It's a path we walk in community, sharing our experiences, supporting each other, and learning from one another. As we connect with others, we expand our understanding of ourselves and our place in the universe. This interconnectedness is essential for our spiritual growth and evolution. We are not alone on this journey.

The journey toward liberating the soul and experiencing its immortality requires courage, commitment, and unwavering faith in our own inner potential. It's a journey of continuous self-discovery and growth, a process of peeling away layers of illusion to uncover the boundless beauty and wisdom within. This process may involve confronting deep-seated fears and insecurities, releasing limiting beliefs, and embracing our authentic selves. But with dedication and perseverance, we can unlock our inner potential and experience the profound joy and freedom that come with living a life aligned with our true nature.

This journey is not a destination; it is a continuous process of unfolding, a constant expansion of awareness and understanding. The true immortality of the soul is not a static state, but a dynamic and evolving expression of consciousness. It is a life lived in harmony with the universe, a life of purpose, meaning, and boundless love. As we walk this path, we embrace not only our own liberation, but also contribute to the liberation of others, creating a ripple effect of peace, compassion, and understanding in the world. The immortality of the soul is not a separate entity, but the echo of our life lived fully, lovingly and in complete connection with the universe.

The Role of Karma and Dharma in Spiritual Growth

The journey towards the immortality of the soul, as we've begun to explore, is not merely a passive acceptance of some ethereal promise, but an active, conscious participation in the unfolding of existence. It demands engagement, understanding, and a profound acceptance of the interwoven tapestry of cause and effect, of action and consequence, which is the very fabric of our experience. This is where the concepts of karma and dharma become crucial, providing a framework for navigating this journey with intention and purpose.

Karma, often misinterpreted as a simplistic system of reward and punishment, is far more nuanced. It's not a cosmic scorekeeper doling out retribution or blessings, but rather a principle of natural consequence, an intrinsic law governing the energetic interplay of our actions and their repercussions. Every thought, word, and deed generates vibrations, ripples in the cosmic ocean of energy, that reverberate outwards, influencing our present and shaping our future. These are not arbitrary judgments; they are the natural unfolding of cause and effect, an echo of our own energetic creations.

Understanding karma involves acknowledging the interconnectedness of all things. Our actions don't exist in isolation; they ripple outwards, affecting not only ourselves but also those around us, and ultimately, the larger cosmic web of existence. A seemingly small act of kindness can have far-reaching consequences, creating a cascade of positive energy that extends beyond our immediate sphere of influence. Conversely, an act of negativity, even a fleeting thought of malice, can create a ripple of disharmony that impacts our lives and the lives of others. This interconnectedness underscores the importance of mindful action, of approaching our interactions with awareness and compassion.

The concept of karma is not meant to instill fear or guilt, but to foster responsibility. It's a call to cultivate awareness of the impact of our actions, not only on a personal level but on the wider world. It encourages us to approach our lives with intention, to consciously choose actions that align with our highest values, leading to a harmonious existence. The focus shouldn't be on avoiding negative consequences, but on cultivating positive intentions and nurturing a compassionate heart. By understanding the ripple effect of our actions, we can actively participate in shaping a more harmonious reality for ourselves and for all beings.

Dharma, on the other hand, speaks to our purpose, our unique contribution to the grand symphony of existence. It's not a pre-ordained destiny, but rather our inherent potential, our individual expression within the cosmic whole. Discovering our dharma is a process of self-discovery, a journey of introspection and exploration. It involves identifying our talents, passions, and values, and aligning our actions with these inherent qualities. Living in accordance with our dharma leads to a life of fulfillment, purpose, and profound satisfaction.

The path to discovering our dharma can be a winding one, filled with challenges and detours. It's a journey of self-reflection, of paying attention to the subtle whispers of our inner voice. It often requires stepping outside our comfort zones, embracing change, and venturing into the unknown. We may find ourselves drawn towards paths that initially seem unconventional, or even challenging. But it's in these moments of uncertainty and growth that we often discover our deepest truths and our most profound purpose. The true path often lies not in ease or comfort, but in facing our fears and embracing our unique capabilities.

Understanding our dharma is essential to our spiritual growth because it provides a sense of direction and meaning. It helps us connect with our deeper purpose, aligning our actions with the larger cosmic plan. When we are living in accordance with our dharma, we experience a sense of flow, a sense of effortless ease and natural harmony. This isn't a passive acceptance of fate, but an active participation in the creative force of the universe, a contribution to the evolution of consciousness itself.

The interplay between karma and dharma is dynamic and ever-evolving. Our actions, governed by the principles of karma, shape our future experiences, while our dharma provides a compass, guiding us toward a life of purpose and fulfillment. Living in alignment with our dharma helps us mitigate negative karma, fostering balance and harmony in our lives. It's not about avoiding challenges or seeking constant happiness, but about navigating life's ups and downs with grace and resilience, understanding that even difficult experiences can contribute to our growth and evolution.

Imagine a river flowing towards the ocean. The river's path, its course, represents our dharma, the natural flow of our individual potential. The rocks, the currents, the eddies along the way, represent the challenges and obstacles we encounter, the consequences of our past actions (karma). While we may encounter rapids and turbulent waters, the overall direction, the ultimate destination, remains the same: the vast and boundless ocean of consciousness. The journey itself is the process of spiritual growth, the refinement of our being, the continuous unfolding of our potential.

Furthermore, the concepts of karma and dharma are intrinsically linked to the concept of reincarnation, a fundamental principle in many spiritual traditions. Karma isn't merely about the consequences of actions in a single lifetime; it extends across multiple lifetimes, creating a continuous cycle of growth and evolution. Each incarnation provides an opportunity to learn from past experiences, to refine our choices, and to move closer towards a state of liberation. The lessons learned, the karmic debts settled, and the progress made in each life contribute to the overall spiritual journey. The soul, in this context, is not a static entity, but a dynamic force, constantly evolving and learning.

This perspective shifts our understanding of suffering and hardship. Challenges and setbacks, often viewed as negative experiences, become opportunities for growth and refinement. They are not punishments, but lessons, opportunities to learn from our mistakes, to refine our choices, and to deepen our compassion. Through these experiences, we develop resilience, wisdom, and a deeper understanding of the interconnectedness of all things.

The journey towards liberation and the immortality of the soul, therefore, becomes a conscious engagement with karma and dharma. It's not about escaping the cycle of birth and death, but about transforming the cycle, about consciously shaping our experiences through mindful action and aligned purpose. By understanding the consequences of our actions and living in harmony with our inner guidance, we move towards a state of liberation, a state of effortless existence, where we are fully integrated into the cosmic flow, living a life of purpose, fulfillment, and ultimately, a life that extends beyond the limitations of the physical form. This is the essence of the immortal soul, not a static entity, but a dynamic expression of consciousness, constantly evolving, learning, and contributing to the beauty and harmony of the universe.

The process of self-discovery, integral to uncovering one's dharma, requires introspection and self-awareness. Meditation practices, as discussed in previous chapters, are invaluable tools in this journey. By quieting the mind and connecting with our inner selves, we gain access to the wisdom and guidance that resides within. This inner wisdom reveals our unique talents, our passions, and our inherent values, leading us towards actions that resonate with our deepest truth and purpose. This is not a passive process, but an active engagement with our inner landscape, a conscious exploration of our potential and our unique contribution to the world.

Furthermore, the practice of compassion, integral to mitigating negative karma and fostering harmonious relationships, is another vital element of this journey. Compassion allows us to see the interconnectedness of all beings, understanding that our actions affect not only ourselves but also others. It encourages us to approach our interactions with empathy and understanding, fostering positive relationships and creating a ripple effect of harmony and well-being. This, in turn, creates a virtuous cycle, reinforcing our dharma and promoting spiritual growth. The cultivation of compassion isn't merely an ethical principle; it's a spiritual practice, a way of aligning ourselves with the inherent goodness and interconnectedness of the universe.

The path towards liberation and the immortality of the soul is not a solitary journey. It's a path shared with others, a journey of connection and mutual support. Engaging with our communities, contributing to the well-being of others, and actively participating in creating a more harmonious world are all integral aspects of our spiritual growth. By extending our compassion and support to those around us, we create a ripple effect of positive energy that benefits not only others but also ourselves. This mutual support system enhances our ability to navigate the challenges of life and to move closer towards our ultimate purpose. The immortality of the soul is not an isolated achievement; it's a reflection of our connection to all beings and our contribution to the well-being of the world.

A State of Pure Awareness

The culmination of our journey towards the immortality of the soul lies in the liberation of the mind – a state of pure awareness, unburdened by the incessant chatter of thoughts, emotions, and the ego's relentless demands. This is not a mere cessation of mental activity, but a transcendence of it, a profound shift in consciousness that allows us to perceive reality with clarity and unwavering presence. It is the unlocking of our true potential, the unveiling of our inherent connection to the divine, the boundless source of all existence.

This state of pure awareness isn't a destination to be reached at some distant point in the future; it's a process, an unfolding, a continuous refinement of our perception and understanding. It's a journey of self-discovery, a peeling away of layers of conditioning and ingrained patterns of thought and behavior that have obscured our true nature. The practice of meditation provides the vehicle for this journey, the pathway to this profound transformation.

Consistent meditation, practiced with dedication and unwavering intention, gradually dissolves the veil of illusion that separates us from our true selves. As we quiet the mind, we begin to experience glimpses of this pure awareness – moments of profound stillness, where the incessant flow of thoughts ceases, and we are left with a sense of boundless peace and clarity. These moments, initially fleeting, become longer and more frequent with continued practice.

The key to unlocking this state lies in cultivating a deep awareness of the present moment. We must learn to observe our thoughts and emotions without judgment, recognizing them as fleeting phenomena that arise and pass away like clouds in the sky. We are not our thoughts; we are the awareness that observes them. This distinction is crucial; it's the cornerstone of mental liberation.

Imagine the mind as a turbulent ocean, its waves representing the constant stream of thoughts and emotions. The goal of meditation is not to suppress these waves, but to learn to observe them from a place of stillness – to become the calm, deep ocean floor beneath the surface. As we cultivate this deep awareness, the turbulent waves gradually subside, revealing the tranquil depths of our being.

This process of observing without judgment is vital. Our tendency is to identify with our thoughts and emotions, to become entangled in their narratives. We label ourselves as "anxious," "angry," or "depressed," allowing these labels to define our sense of self. However, this identification reinforces the cycle of suffering. By observing these emotions without judgment, we begin to disentangle ourselves from their grip, recognizing their impermanent nature.

Regular meditation practice, coupled with mindfulness throughout the day, fosters this non-judgmental observation. Notice your thoughts and emotions as they arise, without clinging to them or resisting them. Simply acknowledge their presence and let them pass. This act of non-attachment is crucial in dissolving the grip of the ego, which thrives on identification with thoughts and emotions.

The practice of Pranayama, the conscious control of breath, is an invaluable tool in achieving this state of pure awareness. By regulating our breath, we regulate the flow of prana, the vital life force energy that permeates our being. Deep, slow, and controlled breathing calms the nervous system, reducing stress and anxiety, creating space for the mind to quieten. Specific breathing techniques, such as alternate nostril breathing (Nadi Shodhana), can further enhance this process, balancing the energies within the body and fostering a state of inner harmony.

Furthermore, cultivating a loving-kindness meditation practice can significantly contribute to the liberation of the mind. By extending feelings of compassion and unconditional love to ourselves and others, we soften the heart, releasing the grip of negativity and resentment. This practice not only fosters inner peace but also strengthens our connection to the divine, the source of boundless love and compassion. It melts away the barriers of self-imposed limitations, unveiling the inherent goodness within ourselves and others.

As we progress on this path, we may encounter moments of resistance. The mind, accustomed to its habitual patterns, may resist the stillness, clinging to its familiar distractions. This is a natural part of the process. It's important to approach these moments with patience and compassion, gently guiding the mind back to the present moment, to the breath, to the awareness of the body's sensations.

The journey towards liberation is not a linear one; it's a process of ebb and flow, of progress and setbacks. There will be moments of profound clarity and peace, followed by moments of distraction and restlessness. The key is to maintain consistency in our practice, to persevere with unwavering determination, and to cultivate a deep sense of self-compassion. Celebrate the moments of stillness, and gently guide yourself back to the path when you stray.

The rewards of this journey are immeasurable. As we achieve liberation of the mind, we experience a profound sense of freedom, a release from the suffering that arises from our identification with the ego. We develop a deeper understanding of our true nature, our inherent connection to the divine, and our potential for infinite growth and expansion. This liberation is not merely a mental state; it's a fundamental shift in consciousness that permeates every aspect of our lives. It transforms our relationships, our work, our interactions with the world, and our understanding of ourselves.

The state of pure awareness is not a passive state; it's a state of active, conscious engagement with life. It's a state of unwavering presence, a deep appreciation for the beauty and wonder of each moment. It allows us to approach challenges with greater clarity, resilience, and compassion. It empowers us to live with greater intention and purpose, to create a life that is meaningful and fulfilling.

This liberation of the mind isn't merely a means to an end; it's the very essence of the path towards the immortality of the soul. As we shed the limitations of the ego, we begin to experience a deeper connection to the divine, to the boundless energy that permeates all existence. This connection transcends the physical body, extending beyond the limitations of time and space, offering a glimpse into the boundless possibilities of the soul's immortal journey.

The practice of meditation is not just a technique; it's a transformation of consciousness. It's a process of self-discovery, a journey into the depths of our being, a rediscovery of our inherent divinity. It's a way to cultivate inner peace, resilience, and compassion, all while opening ourselves to the boundless potential of the soul's journey towards immortality. The path may be challenging at times, but the rewards are beyond measure. The journey to liberation is a journey to the heart of our being, and a journey to the heart of existence itself. It is a journey towards a profound and lasting freedom – the freedom of pure awareness, the gateway to the immortality of the soul. The path is open; the journey awaits. Begin.

Your Spiritual Heaven on Earth

Having explored the profound techniques of meditation and their transformative power on the mind and spirit, we now arrive at the culmination of our journey: living a life of purpose and meaning – your spiritual heaven on earth. This isn't about escaping reality to some ethereal realm, but about transforming our perception of it, imbuing our everyday existence with the depth, richness, and joy that comes from living in alignment with our true selves. The liberation of the mind, as discussed in the previous chapter, paves the way for this profound shift in consciousness. It is the bedrock upon which we build a life not just of longevity, but of lasting significance.

The pursuit of immortality, in the context of this book, is not about an endless physical existence, but about the preservation and expansion of our consciousness, our soul's essence. This preservation extends into the vibrancy of our lives here and now. A life infused with purpose radiates a life force that extends far beyond the constraints of our physical bodies. It is a life lived fully, authentically, and in harmony with the universe.

This profound sense of purpose isn't something that magically appears overnight. It's cultivated, nurtured, and refined through conscious intention and consistent practice. It begins with introspection – a deep dive into our values, passions, and the unique gifts we bring to the world. Ask yourself: What truly ignites my soul? What am I driven to contribute? What legacy do I wish to leave behind? These questions, when contemplated through the lens of meditative awareness, can unlock profound insights into your life's purpose.

The answers may not come easily. The path to self-discovery is often a winding road, filled with moments of clarity and periods of introspection. Embrace the journey, allowing yourself to explore different avenues, to experiment with different paths, and to trust the intuitive wisdom that arises from within. Do not be afraid to deviate from the charted course, to follow the whispers of your heart, even if it leads you down unfamiliar trails. The process itself is as vital as the destination.

Once you begin to grasp your unique purpose, it's crucial to translate that understanding into action. Purpose without action remains a dormant seed, unable to blossom into its full potential. Find ways to integrate your purpose into your daily life, however small or seemingly insignificant they may seem at first. Perhaps it's volunteering your time for a cause you care deeply about, pursuing a creative endeavor, or simply engaging in acts of kindness and compassion. Every step, every conscious choice aligned with your purpose, strengthens the connection to your true self and intensifies your life force.

Cultivating meaningful relationships is equally vital. These connections enrich our lives, providing support, inspiration, and a sense of belonging. Genuine connections, built on mutual respect, empathy, and understanding, nourish our souls and contribute to a sense of wholeness. They help us to move beyond the limitations of the ego and to embrace our interconnectedness with others and the universe. Nurturing these relationships, both personally and professionally, is a crucial aspect of building a life imbued with purpose and meaning.

Living a life of purpose often entails navigating challenges and overcoming obstacles. These difficulties, rather than being seen as roadblocks, should be regarded as opportunities for growth, resilience, and spiritual deepening. Each challenge, when met with courage, mindfulness, and a commitment to learning, contributes to the expansion of our consciousness and strengthens our resolve. The practice of meditation equips us with the tools to navigate these challenges with grace and equanimity.

Remember that our spiritual journey is a continuous process of evolution and transformation. It's not about reaching a fixed destination, but about embracing the journey itself. Embrace the inevitable ups and downs, the moments of exhilaration and the periods of quiet contemplation. It's in the integration of these experiences that we truly grow and evolve. Embrace the ebbs and flows of life as integral aspects of your journey.

The concept of "spiritual heaven on earth" doesn't imply a utopian escape from reality but rather a profound transformation of our perception. It's about creating a life that's rich in meaning, purpose, and authentic connection. It's about recognizing the divine spark within ourselves and radiating that energy out into the world. This is not a passive state of being, but an active engagement with life, fueled by a deep sense of purpose and guided by the wisdom gained through meditation and self-awareness.

This spiritual heaven is not a destination to be reached but a state of being cultivated through the consistent practice of the principles outlined in this book. It's about integrating the practices of meditation, breathwork, and mindful living into the fabric of your everyday life. It's about cultivating inner peace, resilience, and a deep sense of connection with the universe.

As you move forward in your journey, remember to regularly reflect on your progress. Journaling, meditation, or quiet contemplation can provide invaluable insights into your growth and development. Identify any areas where you might need to make adjustments or deepen your practice. Remember that self-compassion is crucial; be patient and kind to yourself as you navigate this transformative process. Don't strive for perfection, instead focus on continuous improvement and progress, even if that is just one small step each day.

Consider creating rituals and routines that support your spiritual practice. This could include setting aside dedicated time each day for meditation, journaling, or mindful movement. Surrounding yourself with inspirational people and resources can also nurture your growth. Engage in activities that uplift and inspire you, whether it's spending time in nature, listening to uplifting music, or connecting with loved ones.

Finally, remember that your spiritual journey is a deeply personal one. There is no one-size-fits-all approach. Trust your intuition, listen to the wisdom of your heart, and create a path that aligns with your unique needs and aspirations. Embrace the process with open arms and allow yourself to be guided by the inner wisdom that resides within you.

The practices and principles discussed in this book provide a framework for achieving spiritual liberation and living a life of purpose and meaning. They are tools to support you on your journey. The responsibility for creating your spiritual heaven on earth lies in your hands. Embrace this responsibility, nurture your potential, and watch your life blossom into a vibrant testament to the enduring power of the human spirit. The path is illuminated; the journey is yours to embark on. Begin. Live a life filled with purpose, meaning, and the enduring grace of your immortal soul. The potential is within you, waiting to be unleashed.

Acknowledgments

This book would not have been possible without the support and guidance of many individuals. First and foremost, I express my deepest gratitude to my teachers and mentors, whose wisdom and unwavering dedication to spiritual practice have profoundly shaped my understanding and approach to meditation. Their patience, insight, and encouragement have been invaluable throughout this journey.

I am also deeply indebted to my family and friends, whose love and support have sustained me during the writing process. Their unwavering belief in my work and their willingness to offer feedback and encouragement have been instrumental to the completion of this book.

A special thank you to [Name of Editor/Agent], whose expertise and guidance were crucial in shaping this manuscript into its final form. Their insightful feedback and dedication to excellence have greatly enhanced the clarity and impact of this work. Finally, I extend my heartfelt gratitude to all those who have shared their personal experiences of meditation with me. Their stories of transformation and healing serve as a testament to the power of this ancient practice and have inspired me immensely.

Appendix

This appendix provides supplementary materials to enhance your meditative practice.

Guided Meditations: [Include links or descriptions to downloadable audio files or scripts for guided meditations corresponding to techniques described in the book.]

Journal Prompts: [Provide a list of journal prompts designed to encourage reflection and deepen the reader's understanding of their spiritual journey, aligning with the themes of the book.]

Resources: [List relevant websites, books, or organizations related to meditation, holistic health, and spiritual development.]

Glossary

Prana: The vital life force energy that flows through the
body.
Chakra: Energy centers within the body.
Mindfulness: The practice of paying attention to the present
moment without judgment.
Trataka: Gaze meditation focusing on a single point.
Karma: The principle of cause and effect.
Dharma: One's purpose or path in life.
Telomeres: Protective caps on chromosomes, linked to
aging and longevity.

References

[List of scientific studies, books, articles, and other sources cited throughout the book, formatted according to a consistent citation style, such as APA or MLA.]

Author Biography

[Author Name] is a [brief description of author's credentials and experience related to meditation, spirituality, and holistic well-being]. [He/She/They] have dedicated [number] years to the study and practice of meditation, integrating these principles into [his/her/their] daily life. [Author Name]'s passion lies in sharing the transformative power of meditation with others, empowering them to live more fulfilling, meaningful, and spiritually enriched lives. [He/She/They] have [mention any relevant achievements, such as leading workshops, retreats, or previous publications]. [Author Name] believes that the path to immortality of the soul lies not in extending physical lifespan, but in cultivating inner peace, wisdom, and a deep connection with the divine.